How Caregiving Affects Development

How Caregiving Affects Development

PSYCHOLOGICAL IMPLICATIONS *for* CHILD, ADOLESCENT, *and* ADULT CAREGIVERS

EDITED BY

Kim Shifren

AMERICAN PSYCHOLOGICAL ASSOCIATION
WASHINGTON, DC

Published by
American Psychological Association
750 First Street, NE
Washington, DC 20002
www.apa.org

To order
APA Order Department
P.O. Box 92984
Washington, DC 20090-2984
Tel: (800) 374-2721; Direct: (202) 336-5510
Fax: (202) 336-5502; TDD/TTY: (202) 336-6123
Online: www.apa.org/books/
E-mail: order@apa.org

In the U.K., Europe, Africa, and the Middle East, copies may be ordered from
American Psychological Association
3 Henrietta Street
Covent Garden, London
WC2E 8LU England

Typeset in Minion by Circle Graphics, Columbia, MD

Printer: Edwards Brothers, Inc., Ann Arbor, MI
Cover Designer: Berg Design, Albany, NY
Technical/Production Editor: Harriet Kaplan

The opinions and statements published are the responsibility of the authors, and such opinions and statements do not necessarily represent the policies of the American Psychological Association.

Library of Congress Cataloging-in-Publication Data

How caregiving affects development : psychological implications for child, adolescent, and adult caregivers / edited by Kim Shifren. — 1st ed.
    p. cm.
  Includes bibliographical references and index.
  ISBN-13: 978-1-4338-0393-2
  ISBN-10: 1-4338-0393-3
  1. Developmental psychology. 2. Caregivers. I. Shifren, Kim.

  BF713.H69 2009
  155.9'24—dc22
                              2008010791

British Library Cataloguing-in-Publication Data
A CIP record is available from the British Library.

Printed in the United States of America
First Edition

Contents

Contributors

Audie A. Atienza, National Cancer Institute, Bethesda, MD

Laurie J. Bauman, Albert Einstein College of Medicine, Bronx, NY

Rebecca Berman, CJE Senior Life, Chicago, IL

Maureen Blankemeyer, Kent State University, Kent, OH

Mary Dellmann-Jenkins, Kent State University, Kent, OH

Melissa M. Franks, Purdue University, West Lafayette, IN

Ivy Gamble, New York, NY

Eric A. Goedereis, West Virginia University, Morgantown

Lynn M. Martire, University of Pittsburgh School of Medicine, Pittsburgh, PA

Tina R. Norton, Clarkson University, Potsdam, NY

Julie Hicks Patrick, West Virginia University, Morgantown

Kim Shifren, Towson University, Towson, MD

Ellen Johnson Silver, Albert Einstein College of Medicine, Bronx, NY

Connie Siskowski, Volunteers for the Homebound and Family Caregivers, Inc., Boca Raton, FL

Catherine H. Stein, Bowling Green State University, Bowling Green, OH

Mary Ann Parris Stephens, Kent State University, Kent, OH

How Caregiving
Affects Development

Introduction: A Life Span Perspective on Caregivers

Kim Shifren

Caregiving is a national issue that continues to increase in importance over time. People are living longer than ever before, and diseases that once meant a shorter life span now have available treatments. Instead of shorter life spans, individuals may be living with chronic illnesses and disabilities that require ongoing care (Verbrugge, 1989). Many adult caregivers provide informal unpaid care to adults with chronic illnesses and disabilities. The mental and physical health of caregivers, their social support system, coping strategies, and levels of stress and burden remain a major focus of research, as evidenced by a number of recent literature reviews and meta-analyses (e.g., Haley, 2003; Pinquart & Sörensen, 2003, 2005; Vitaliano, Zhang, & Scanlan, 2003). The positive aspects of caregiving experiences are receiving increased attention as well (Beach, 1997; Boerner, Schulz, & Horowitz, 2004; Hooker, Monahan, Bowman, Frazier, & Shifren, 1998; Roff et al. 2004). Some caregivers derive positive meaning from the caregiving role (Beach, 1997), whereas others experience both positive and negative affect (Robertson, Zarit, Duncan, Rovine, & Femia, 2007). Some caregivers even show stability and increases in their level of optimism over time (Shifren & Hooker, 1995).

Most caregiving research in the United States has been focused on adult caregivers, especially middle-aged (40s to early 60s) and older adult (65 and over) caregivers (Hooker et al., 1998; Vitaliano et al., 2003). This is due in part to the large number of adult caregivers in this country.

Approximately 44.4 million adults (people ages 18 and older) provide unpaid care to another adult in the United States (National Alliance for Caregiving & the American Association of Retired Persons, 2004). However, recent literature shows that caregiving occurs across the life span from childhood through older adulthood (Beach, 1997; Dellmann-Jenkins & Brittain, 2003; Gates & Lackey, 1998; Hooker, Manoogian-O'Dell, Monahan, Frazier, & Shifren, 2000; Lackey & Gates, 2001; Levine et al., 2005; Nolen-Hoeksema & Ahrens, 2002; Shifren & Kachorek, 2003). In fact, between 1.3 million and 1.4 million individuals between ages 8 and 18 years could be considered caregivers, according to the first national U.S. survey on the prevalence of this demographic (Hunt, Levine, & Naiditch, 2005).

Because caregiving is not solely an adult activity, it is useful to study caregiving experiences from a life span development perspective that includes both the youngest caregivers (people in early childhood) and older adult caregivers. The life span development perspective, that is, the view that development is a lifelong process from conception to death, takes into account the overall development of caregivers' behaviors as a dynamic process involving both gains and losses throughout the life span (Baltes, Staudinger, & Lindenberger, 1999). Becoming a caregiver at any point in the life span will affect the caregiver's current and future development.

A life span development perspective is the overarching theme of this book. Chapter authors discuss their research findings on caregivers within a life span development framework. Each chapter includes information on the tasks that are associated with normal development and the ongoing interaction between the caregiving role and these developmental tasks for specific caregiver samples. Whenever research has included a comparison group of noncaregivers, a discussion is provided comparing caregiver with noncaregiver development.

The first part of this chapter provides background on the relevant principles of life span development. The second part discusses the overarching theme of the book, caregiving from a life span perspective. Specific developmental principles for each age group are briefly discussed within the life span development framework, and the possible effects of caregiving at each developmental period are examined. For each developmental period there is a brief description of the chapter on caregivers for that part of the life span.

KEY PRINCIPLES OF LIFE SPAN DEVELOPMENT

Much of the caregiving literature could be enhanced with the use of the life span development approach. The key principles of this perspective include the ideas that (a) development is lifelong, (b) development is dependent on history and context, (c) development is multidimensional and multidirectional, and (d) development is pliable (Baltes, 1987; Baltes, Lindenberger, & Staudinger, 1998).

Development Is Lifelong

Development occurs throughout the life span, from conception to death, and earlier periods affect current and future development. Each period of development is conceptualized as being equally important (Baltes et al., 1998). Caregiving at any point in the life span will affect the development of the caregiver. For example, caregiving in middle childhood can affect school performance and attendance, which may in turn affect future education (Dearden & Becker, 1999). Most researchers are aware of this, even if they do not address this issue in their own work.

Development Is Dependent on History and Context

Human beings develop at specific times and places and both influence and are affected by historical periods in which they live (e.g., the period following the September 11th attacks on the United States, the Great Depression).[1] With caregiving, as with other human activities, it is important to consider how caregiving experiences differ because of the time in history in which they take place. One example is the fact that at different historical periods there has been more or less financial support and formal support outside the home for informal caregivers. In other words,

---

[1] Elder (1974) used a similar line of reasoning in his work on what he termed "life course trajectory." He discussed the ways in which different points of a person's life are connected (Elder, George, & Shanahan, 1996).

some caregivers may have had no financial help from government, state, or local resources. Thus, the experiences of being a caregiver from a particular cohort, not just of a particular age group, can be quite different.

People develop within specific contexts and influence and are affected by these contexts. For example, caregivers who live and care for others in impoverished environments will have caregiving experiences much different from those with more available resources. "An impoverished environment" could refer to financial difficulties but could also describe a situation in which a family has lost most relatives and is socially isolated. That is, individuals may provide caregiving in a context that is impoverished both financially and socially.

Bronfenbrenner (1986) argued that children's development is strongly influenced by multiple contexts, including the family, school, peer group, and neighborhood and community. How might dynamic change in the context of the family affect individuals over time? For caregivers, there may be an accelerated life course, much like that suggested for inner-city minority youth (Burton, Obeidallah, & Allison, 1996). Individuals may need to begin emotional autonomy, making independent decisions (Arnett, 2000; Papalia, Olds, & Feldman, 2007) about finances and health care at a much younger age than is typical for these kinds of decisions.

Development Is Multidimensional and Multidirectional

Human development involves both growth and decline along multiple dimensions, including physical, cognitive, and psychosocial development, and occurs throughout the life span. For example, older adults may learn to minimize loss in some cognitive functioning (e.g., source memory) by using expertise in specific domains (Jastrzembski, Charness, & Vasyukova, 2006). Also, we influence other people and our environment, and other people and the environment can affect us too. Unfortunately, very young caregivers may miss out on growth opportunities in some of these dimensions, because they may have limited time available to experience social interactions or they are missing school (Siskowski, 2006). Older adult caregivers may need to compensate for declines in their own physical abilities when helping to move care recipients or declines in memory capacity when giving care recipients medications. In terms of multidirectionality, people influence other people and their environment, and vice versa. For example, rather than relationships being strictly unidirectional from the caregiver to the care recipient, relations between caregivers and care receivers involve an ongoing dynamic interaction between them.

Development Is Pliable

People are *pliable*—able to adapt to changing environments. The caregiving role can change quickly, especially when it involves caring for individuals with diseases like Alzheimer's. It can be rewarding to caregivers to know that they can handle the changes taking place and adapt accordingly (Beach, 1997).

Importance of Life Span Principles in Research on Caregiving

The life span principles discussed above are important for understanding the similarities and differences in experiences of caregivers from different parts of the life span. The historical and contextual changes that have taken place in the United States help guide research questions. For example, why would grandparent caregivers be taking on full-time caregiver roles for their grandchildren with more frequency than ever before? Changes in demographics, nutrition, and medicine have led to an increase in caregiving responsibilities for grandparents (Davies & Williams, 2002). Other life span principles can guide further research questions. One principle, that development is multidirectional, could guide questions on the attachment relation between grandparents and grandchildren. How does being a full-time grandparent caregiver affect attachment with their grandchildren? These are just two examples of the many interesting questions that can be developed for research on caregiving on the basis of the life span principles.

CAREGIVING FROM A LIFE SPAN DEVELOPMENT FRAMEWORK

The life span perspective can provide a broader framework for thinking about caregiving research questions. For example, it is clear from much research that significant changes in physical health can occur in older adult caregivers as a result of the caregiving experience, including elevated stress hormones, increased risk for hypertension and diabetes, and immune system risks such as decreased antibody production (Vitaliano et al. 2003).

As for younger caregivers, it is known that there are physical health threats to the children and adolescents involved in early caregiving, such as the risk of injury resulting from poor techniques used to lift a parent in and out of beds, chairs, and bathroom facilities (Dearden & Becker, 1999; Gates & Lackey, 1998), but it is not clear how the immune systems of young caregivers are affected or the level of stress hormones present that may put them at risk for later disease development. Therefore, from a life span perspective, the long-term effects of early caregiving on adult physical health is an important question for future research on caregivers.

Life span principles, such as the idea that development is dependent on context and that development is multidimensional, can guide research questions on caregiving. To better appreciate the wide variety of questions one can ask, one first must understand what constitutes normal development in different domains. Therefore, an important goal for this chapter is to include discussion of the cognitive, physical, and psychosocial domains of development over the life span.

The following discussion addresses a number of the developmental changes that occur in each period of the life span and integrates a brief discussion of the chapters in this book that address caregiving within specific developmental periods. The multidimensional nature of development (i.e., changes in physical, cognitive, and psychosocial development) as well as the importance of context are incorporated into the discussion where appropriate.

Child Caregivers and Life Span Development

Although caregiving at any age may be a nonnormative event (Hooker et al., 1998), it may be more likely to be perceived as nonnormative for child caregivers. For example, in the United States, it is not expected that children assist adults with bathing and dressing. As you will read in chapter 1 of this volume, however, children are indeed providing hands-on care involving these kinds of activities. Children as young as 5 years have provided primary care for a parent or adult relative (Gates & Lackey, 1998; Shifren & Kachorek, 2003). No study has been done at this time to determine the specific portion of the U.S. population that is between 5 and 10 years old and providing hands-on care to a parent or adult relative. The first national U.S. survey examined individuals 8 to 18 years old and found that 3 in 10 child caregivers are 8 to 11 years old, with 38% ages 12 to 15 and 31% ages 16 to 18 years old (Levine et al., 2005). Lackey and Gates (2001) found that almost one half of their sample ($n = 51$) began caregiving at or before age 10. In a recent study (Shifren, 2008), I found that almost one third of my sample ($n = 38$) began caregiving (i.e., bathing, dressing) for a parent at or before age 10.

Normal cognitive development in children from ages 3 to 6 requires developmental tasks that enable children to gain insight into their own mental processes, learn to use symbols, learn to identify similarities and differences in categories of people and objects, and learn social skills. Although there is some evidence that young children can understand others' viewpoints, such understanding does not appear to occur for abstract concepts like the famous three mountain task (Piaget & Inhelder, 1967), in which a child is placed at a table with models of three mountains, a doll is placed on a chair at the opposite side of the table from the child, and the child is asked to describe what the doll sees from its side of the table. Young children generally give their own viewpoint rather than the view of the doll, indicating that the child cannot understand another person's view.

The key principle of life span development—that development is dependent on context—is useful when discussing cognitive development in child caregivers. On the one hand, child caregivers may miss out on preschool and kindergarten environments that might stimulate cognitive abilities through the use of creative activities designed to help children learn verbal and math skills. On the other hand, care recipients who are physically but not mentally incapacitated may be able to provide more attention to their child caregivers by, for example, engaging in interactive games with them (even from bed).

Physical development in children from 3 to 6 years old coincides with learning basic tasks of daily living that require the development of fine and gross motor skills, such as dressing, bathing themselves, and brushing their teeth correctly. Children in this age category who are caregivers may be helping adults walk up and down stairs and dress themselves when the children are just beginning to demonstrate complete independence in these same tasks (Dearden & Becker, 1999).

With regard to psychosocial development, early childhood is a time when children are taking the first steps in learning to understand and regulate their emotions. Caregiving for a parent or adult relative may affect their ability to maintain a healthy emotional relationship with the care recipient. Some young children who provide caregiving to a parent may be more resilient to stressors from the caregiving situation than others, similar to children who are resilient to risks in impoverished backgrounds (Garmezy, 1993; Masten et al., 1995, 1999). Impoverished backgrounds could indicate low socioeconomic status that may place children within communities of high violence or drugs. However, an impoverished background may also have to do with the lack of a parental figure, placement in foster care, or living with a mentally impaired parent (Papalia et al., 2007). These individuals may not show health problems or relationship issues in adulthood. Others, however, may not be resilient in the face of such obstacles to healthy development.

The literature on risk and resilience stresses the importance for children to receive both nurturance and supervision from parents if the children are going to be resilient (Tiet et al., 1998). However, a parent may become unable to provide an environment for the child that includes the kinds of nurturance and supervision that would help child development. Consequently, some children and adolescents may lose an important protective factor (i.e., family support) that can help them be resilient in the face of obstacles (Garmezy, 1993). This would be especially true for children in single-parent families in which that parent becomes unable to care for him- or herself, let alone the child.

There may be important individual differences in children that help some deal with caregiving in a positive way whereas others do not. Adult caregiving research includes individual difference variables such as gender (for a review, see Yee & Schulz, 2000) and personality (Hooker et al., 1998).

To take the variable of personality as an example, researchers have demonstrated that personality characteristics can act as filters that influence individuals' perceptions of symptoms and health decisions (Hooker, Frazier, & Monahan, 1994). Personality can influence how caregivers perceive ambiguous situations like the caregiving environment and how well caregivers can detect subtle differences in care recipients' behaviors and health. This is because personality influences where a caregiver will focus his or her attention, including selective attention for positive or negative information (Smith & Rhodewalt, 1986). Personality can influence how much caregivers use information that has been provided for the care recipient's health care when making decisions. Among child caregivers, individual differences in personality will affect how care recipients' needs are handled and how child caregivers feel about their relationship with the care recipient.

Early caregiving may, for some individuals, be a truly thankless job. Some child caregivers perceive their tasks (e.g., bathing a grandparent) as more demanding than the care recipient believes the tasks to be (Gates & Lackey, 1998; Lackey & Gates, 1997). This inconsistency in the perception of task demands can be both frustrating and harmful for the child caregiver. Individuals who do not perceive a child as performing demanding tasks may be uncooperative and unappreciative of such efforts.

During middle childhood (i.e., from 7 to 10 years; Papalia et al., 2007), cognitive development includes improvement in understanding spatial relationships (e.g., memory for routes and landmarks). Older children can use symbols better than younger children (e.g., multiplication and division) and can categorize things better (e.g., arrange objects according to different dimensions; Papalia et al., 2007). Older children can use *inductive reasoning*, which is the ability to draw conclusions about members of a class of people, objects, or events. For instance, if my dog barks, and Mary's dog barks, all dogs must bark. There is also evidence of *deductive reasoning*, a general premise about a class of people, objects, or events, and application of this statement to certain members of the class (Galotti, Komatsu, & Voelz, 1997). All people sneeze, and Kevin is a person. Therefore, Kevin can sneeze. Learning these kinds of cognitive tasks takes ongoing interaction with people and objects. Perhaps taking on the caregiving role in middle childhood can affect children's ability to draw conclusions about classes of people, objects, or events. This has not yet been studied, but a comparison of caregivers with noncaregivers on specific inductive and deductive reasoning tasks would be informative.

In the United States, researchers have found that early caregiving can disrupt school attendance, test performance, and time for social interactions with others (Lackey & Gates, 2001; Siskowski, 2006). Children who are not exposed to such activities because they are missing too much school will suffer in their cognitive development, particularly in middle childhood, when they should be focused on increasing their cognitive and social skills in an academic setting.

The physical development of those in middle childhood includes continual development of the small and large muscles in the body, which allows older children to run faster, jump farther, lift heavier objects, write, tie shoe laces, and better manipulate small objects (like medicine bottles) than younger children (Papalia et al., 2007). Improved control of gross and fine motor movement is helpful to older child caregivers in providing physical support to care recipients, such as in assisting with bathroom activities and opening medicine bottles.

Psychosocial development in middle childhood also involves developing social skills. Peer perceptions greatly influence children in this period, in particular, their self-esteem. In fact, peer relations during middle childhood are strong predictors of how well-adjusted individuals will be in adolescence and adulthood (Masten & Coatsworth, 1998).

The ability to develop and use social skills may be affected by the caregiving role. Any spare time a child has may go to schoolwork, household tasks, or continued caregiving responsibilities (Dearden & Becker, 1999;

Lackey & Gates, 2001; Siskowski, 2006). This could lead to negative mental health consequences for child caregivers during childhood or by the time they reach adulthood. For example, the little research available on young caregivers in the United States indicates that some individuals are at risk for depressive symptoms during childhood (Hunt et al., 2005) and that some report depressive symptoms by adulthood (Shifren & Kachorek, 2003).

Although no early caregiver study has focused on individuals between the ages of 3 and 6 years, some studies have included child and adolescent caregivers who are a bit older. One such study of interest is presented in chapter 1 of this book, which provides a cutting-edge discussion of individuals who have begun caregiving for a parent or adult relative in middle childhood and adolescence. Specifically, the authors discuss their work on individuals in middle childhood and early to midadolescence (children ages 8 to 16) who care for parents with HIV/AIDS in New York City. Their work provides information on the mothers who are ill and the children's caregiving responsibilities, and it compares these mothers and children with a group of healthy mothers and their children. The authors examine the impact of caregiving on child and adolescent well-being. They also assess their samples for age and gender differences in caregiving responsibilities and address some key principles of life span development—development is dependent on context and is multidimensional—with a focus on psychosocial development. Some developmental concepts discussed in their chapter include autonomy, identity formation, self-esteem, parentification, and role reversal.

Adolescent Caregivers and Life Span Development

In traditional developmental literature, individuals from 12 to 18 years old are considered adolescents (Erikson, 1968). Most young caregivers are in early to mid adolescence when they begin caregiving for a parent (Dearden & Becker, 1999; Gates & Lackey, 1998; Shifren & Kachorek, 2003). All adolescents undergo changes in cognition, physical development, and psychosocial development. These changes will be affected by the caregiving role, so the life span development perspective is a useful one from which to examine these individuals.

Cognitive development in adolescence is characterized by beginning to think abstractly and idealistically as formal operational thought emerges (Harter, 1990). Obviously, idealistic thinking is likely to involve adolescents contemplating life as noncaregiving adolescents, especially when the caregiver role is a negative one. Adolescents who find positive benefits from the caregiving role may contemplate life with future opportunities to provide care for others. Perhaps they will select professions that involve giving care to others or even choose friendships that involve giving much emotional support to a friend who is needy.

Physical development in adolescence may have an ongoing interaction with the caregiving role because changes occur in bones, muscles, and hormones during puberty. The life span development theory principle that development is dependent on history is particularly important with regard to puberty. During the past 100 years or so, in the United States and in other countries, the age of puberty has become younger, and thus people are reaching sexual maturity and adult height and weight at an earlier age than people in previous times (Papalia et al., 2007).

Some changes during adolescence (which, as noted, are taking place earlier than in a previous time in history) may be beneficial for helping care recipients with activities of daily living (ADLs), such as bigger and stronger muscles. Other changes may not be helpful for the caregiving role. Many adolescents, particularly girls, are not happy with their body image as their body changes in shape and size. Dissatisfaction with one's body is associated with the onset of mental health problems such as eating disorders (Shifren, Furnham, & Bauserman, 1998). Adolescents who are already dealing with challenges of the caregiving role may have further stressors from these pubertal changes.

Identity development in adolescence is an important psychosocial developmental task (Erikson, 1963). *Identity development* involves contemplation and decision making about future education goals, career trajectories, relationships, sexuality, and other aspects of the self. Adolescent caregivers may become foreclosed in identity status as a coping strategy. Adolescents who are foreclosed in their identity do not contemplate a variety of options to choose from with regard to careers, relationships, and so on. Instead, they tend to base their identity on a more narrow view of themselves, such as how they are currently perceived or viewed by others and/or by their current experiences. Others' expectations of them may narrow the choices they see for themselves in the future. For example, individuals who survive childhood cancer are more foreclosed in identity status as adolescents than teens who have not had cancer (Madan-Swain, Brown, & Foster, 2000). It has been suggested that foreclosure of identity helps the individual deal with a highly stressful situation (Madan-Swain et al., 2000). This may be likely to happen to adolescents who provide early caregiving for a parent. On the one hand, foreclosed identity could be positive for some adolescent caregivers because they may focus on educational experiences and goals toward achieving future caregiving roles as nurses, doctors, or researchers to eliminate the disease that has affected their parent. For example, if an adolescent has a parent with heart disease, then that adolescent might pursue education and career goals related to becoming a cardiologist. On the other hand, a foreclosed identity could be negative for an adolescent caregiver who has less time to focus on school because he or she may feel that future educational goals are limited and might feel compelled to stay close to home rather than going to a college that fits his or her needs. Beach (1997) suggested that the positive meaning derived in adolescent caregivers' roles could lead to more identity exploration rather than less.

Because little research is available on adolescent caregivers, some issues discussed here have not been studied but certainly warrant attention. Chapter 1 of this volume focuses on the parentification of caregivers in middle childhood and adolescence and the effects of the caregiving role on their well-being. However, the authors do not discuss the effects of caregiving on education and school performance. Because education is an important part of the adolescent period of development, it is useful to look at research that does deal with this topic. Chapter 2 of this volume provides information on adolescents who have begun caregiving for a parent or adult relative during their adolescence from Siskowski's research on the What Works Survey for Palm Beach County, Florida. Specifically, Siskowski discusses the number of adolescents who view themselves as young caregivers and the effects of the caregiving role on their school attendance and performance. This study is the first large sample of young caregivers (sixth, seventh, and eighth graders) in the United States that focuses on education and school attendance. In her discussion, Siskowski addresses aspects of the second principle of life span development—development is dependent on context. Siskowski covers aspects of psychosocial development, including identity development and feelings of self-worth, with some discussion of possible differences between caregivers and noncaregivers where such research has been conducted.

Emerging Adult Caregivers and Life Span Development

The concept of emerging adulthood (ages 18 to 25) is relatively new within the field of developmental psychology. Although some researchers studied and promoted this concept as a new period of development (for a review, see Arnett, 2000), most human development textbooks do not include chapters on emerging adulthood (e.g., Papalia et al., 2007).

One feature of cognitive development during emerging adulthood is that individuals begin to think in more relativistic terms as postformal thought develops (Labouvie-Vief, 1998; Sinnott, 1998). Compared with adolescents, people in their early 20s have greater recognition and inclusion of practical limits in logical thinking. Individuals begin to understand how social factors and factors unique to specific situations like caregiving need to be considered when contemplating how to deal with life problems. Emerging adult caregivers may understand that problems (e.g., caregiving) have no clear solutions and that two opposing views may both have merit (Basseches, 1984, 1989). The different levels of cognitive development between adolescence and emerging adulthood can be crucial to understanding developmental differences in the caregiving experience. Individuals in emerging adulthood may be less likely to become resentful or depressed in a caregiving situation than an adolescent caregiver. Because no study has yet been done to compare adolescent and emerging adult caregivers on these variables, this idea is currently strictly speculative.

Emerging adulthood has come to be considered the main time for identity development, which historically was viewed as the task for adolescent development (Arnett, 1998, 2000; Shifren, Furnham, & Bauserman, 2003). Today's typical 18- to 25-year-olds explore more roles, have more varied living situations, and experience more changes in their world views than in any other period in the life span (Goldscheider & Goldscheider, 1994). Emerging adulthood is a time when individuals are most likely to explore their world for a variety of new experiences. For example, many emerging adults live on their own for the first time. This allows the opportunity to experiment with health-related behaviors such as drinking alcohol and sexual activities, which were possibly explored only briefly during adolescence, and to test aspects of their personality without the presence of parental supervision (Greene, Wheatley, & Aldava, 1992). Many of these individuals pursue college or jobs for the first time (Arnett, 2000). Those who are caregivers at this stage of life may not be able to explore these options because of the limitations resulting from their caregiving role (Lackey & Gates, 2001; Levine et al., 2005). Those who were caregivers in childhood and adolescence and who had particularly negative early caregiving experiences may delay marriage and family or decide not to get married and have children once they reach emerging adulthood. Dellmann-Jenkins, Blankemeyer, and Pinkard (2001) found that taking on the caregiving role may make individuals postpone marriage.

When an individual is beginning to contemplate his or her future, the effects of early caregiving experiences may influence perceptions about health-related possible selves (Hooker, 1992) and occupational selves (Kerpelman, Shoffner, & Ross-Griffin, 2002). Research on the different selves generally involves individuals contemplating and writing down potential views of themselves that could occur in the future. For *health-related possible selves*, individuals may write down a list of qualities that will make them healthy in the future, like strong muscles, and/or aspects of themselves that might decline, such as cognitive impairment or organ failure. When individuals discuss *occupational selves*, they are generally describing possible careers they see themselves taking on in the future. Taking on the responsibility of primary caregiving for a parent at an early age may have profound effects on adult relationships because the caregiving role includes a strong emphasis on family cohesion (Beach, 1997). Increased family cohesion may result in less time for the emerging adult to experience the exploration of self. This may inhibit his or her ability to form an identity; consequently, the formation of intimate adult relationships may be difficult. This is another issue that requires further study.

A retrospective study on 38 individuals who provided care for their parents during childhood and adolescence shows an association between family relations and adult support (Shifren, 2008). *Family relations* refers to the relation between parents and children the first 16 years of life, as defined on the instrument used in this study. *Adult support* refers to perceived support from family and friends in adulthood. This study also found that a father's relationship with his young caregiver was significantly related to the caregivers' adult social system. Specifically, the more warmth and caring that the father was reported to have shown toward the young caregiver during the first 16 years of the child's life, the more perceived tangible support available to the young caregiver in adulthood. Warmth from fathers during the first 16 years of life is also associated with reports of larger numbers of relatives and friends available to provide support to young caregivers in adulthood.

Some researchers have argued that social structures that require early jobs or educational choices do not provide the optimal context for identity development in emerging adulthood (Danielsen, Lorem, & Kroger, 2000). If the early caregiving experience could be considered similar to taking on an early job, then it is likely that identity development may be affected in a similar way. Early caregiving might even be considered a sociocultural variable that is a barrier to ego identity formation (Yoder, 2000). How might less time for identity development affect later stages of development? Stein et al. (1998) found that filial obligation is expressed more strongly in emerging adults than in people of middle age (36 to 60 years old). This obligation may be even more strongly felt by children and adolescents who have not completed tasks of development, such as autonomy with regard to both emotional and financial needs (Arnett, 2000; Papalia, et al., 2007). Some researchers have speculated that caregiving can lead to more identity exploration rather than less (Beach, 1997), so caution is warranted on this issue. Some prior research shows that adolescents may become foreclosed in identity when in stressful situations like dealing with cancer (Madan-Swain et al., 2000). Perhaps a study with caregiving and noncaregiving samples of adolescents that examines their identity development would provide important answers to questions on their identity development.

Two chapters in this book compare caregivers from different developmental periods. Chapter 3 addresses filial responsibility in emerging adult and young adult (26- to 40-year-old) caregivers. *Filial responsibility* is defined in chapter 3 as an individual's willingness to care for parents or older relatives for no monetary gain. The authors present major developmental tasks of emerging and young adulthood, which include establishing independence from family of origin (*differentiation*), building intimate relationships, and developing economic independence, and they discuss how caregiving may affect these tasks. Their chapter integrates findings from their research on emerging and young adult caregivers. Chapter 4 (discussed in more detail in the "Young Adult Caregivers and Life Span Development" section that follows) provides a comparison of young and middle-aged adult caregivers on the role of felt obligation in parental caregiving. The author also assesses felt obligation in older adult caregivers.

Young Adult Caregivers and Life Span Development

As stated previously, the concept of emerging adulthood is relatively new to the field of developmental psychology. Many researchers prefer to use developmental labels for individuals in their late teens and early 20s that reflect the traditional view of life span development. In most textbooks about the stages of the life span, *young adulthood* refers to individuals in their early 20s to early 40s (Papalia et al., 2007). Chapter 4 of this volume includes individuals who could be labeled *emerging adults.* However, the author has chosen to discuss individuals in their late teens and early twenties as *young adults*, so her choice of label is retained, even though it differs from the terminology used in chapter 3 of this volume.[2]

Cognitive development of young adults is similar to that of emerging adults. In the beginning of young adulthood (i.e., the emerging adult age range of 18 to 25 years), individuals begin to think in more relativistic terms as postformal thought develops (Labouvie-Vief, 1998; Sinnott,

---

[2] The debate about these labels in developmental psychology is not the focus of this book, but I certainly hope it will encourage discussion of this important idea.

1998). As stated in the previous section, when people reach their early 20s, thinking involves greater recognition and inclusion of practical limits to logical thinking than in adolescence. Much like emerging adults, those in the beginning of young adulthood may understand that problems (e.g., caregiving) have no clear solutions and that two opposing views may both have merit. By the middle and end of young adulthood (30s to early 40s), individuals have had more time to think about various issues and they may have a better ability to recognize that more than one solution to a problem can be correct. Young adult caregivers should feel less stress when making caregiving decisions than child, adolescent, or emerging adult caregivers because their life experiences have allowed them more time to contemplate a variety of choices or solutions to problems that come up in caregiving, especially medical decisions.

Psychosocial development in young adulthood shows important changes from childhood, adolescence, and emerging adulthood. Arnett (2000) argued that young adulthood is distinct from emerging adulthood because individuals in young adulthood show more stability in many aspects of identity development, including work, family, and personal relationships, than individuals in emerging adulthood. What about young adult caregivers? Do they spend more time contemplating further education, full-time jobs, and possible relationships leading to marriage and families of their own as suggested in the literature (Arnett, 2000)? Again, if these individuals have too many caregiving responsibilities, they may be unable to pursue some or all of these developmental tasks. Some young adult caregivers may hesitate to pursue relationships leading to marriage and family. They may view relationships as likely to lead to additional caregiving roles and wish to avoid any situation that would create such roles. However, other young adult caregivers may thrive on caregiving roles, and they may seek additional relationships that could lead to further caregiving, such as providing emotional support or physical assistance to needy friends and family. This may be especially true for those who experience many aspects of caregiving as positive.

The same thinking could affect the types of jobs that young adult caregivers pursue. Individuals who experience caregiving as positive may pursue similar work. Those who find the caregiving role stressful and burdensome, on the other hand, will likely avoid careers that involve help-ing others.

Young adult caregivers may have young families of their own, with children in infancy, preschool, and elementary school whom they must care for while simultaneously filling the role of caregiver for adult relatives like parents or grandparents. This segment of the "sandwich generation" may have issues different from those of the middle adult caregiver for older relatives with teenaged children living at home. Infants and young children are learning how to walk, talk, feed themselves, dress themselves, use the toilet, read, write, and use numbers (Papalia et al., 2007). Young adult caregivers with young children need to figure out how to juggle all the usual child caregiving tasks while performing similar ADLs (e.g., dressing, bathing) for their own parents or other adult relatives.

Chapter 4 provides a comparison of felt obligation for three different developmental periods. In one study, the author compares young adults (average age of 19 years) with middle-aged adults (average age of 45 years) on felt obligation toward their parents. In a separate study, she investigates felt obligation in older adults (average age of 57 years) toward their eld-erly parents (in their 80s). *Felt obligation* is defined by the author as expec-tations for behavior as viewed within personal relationships among family members across the life span (see also Stein et al., 1998). She studies felt obligation as a set of duties that happens within adults' continual relation-ships with their parents. Using the life span framework, she discusses how felt obligation is multidimensional and how obligation within family is also dependent on history and context. She presents the differences between filial responsibility as discussed in chapter 3 of this volume and felt obligation research presented in her own chapter.

Middle Adult Caregivers and Life Span Development

Middle adulthood is considered the period of life that includes individu-als from their mid-40s to their early 60s (Papalia et al., 2007). What kinds of changes are taking place in the lives of middle adult caregivers? Their lives are complex, with multiple competing demands (Lachman, 2004). Demands on middle adult caregivers include child rearing; part- and full-time jobs; family relationships; work- and community-related activities; and last, but certainly not least, caregiving for one or both parents or other adult relatives (Lachman & James, 1997; Soederberg Miller & Lachman, 2000).

While juggling multiple responsibilities, middle adult caregivers also experience some changes in their cognitive abilities. Luckily most declines are small, and most cognitive abilities remain intact and can even improve with time. Cognitive performance appears to be at its peak in middle age for higher order abilities such as inductive reasoning and vocabulary (Schaie, 1996; Willis & Schaie, 1999), but perceptual speed shows some decline (Schaie, 1996; Soederberg Miller & Lachman, 2000). Even someone whose cognition is at its highest performance level will be tested to the limit with so many demands competing for his or her attention. It would not be surprising if individuals in middle adulthood who become part of the "sandwich generation" often feel overwhelmed and unable to focus attention on the tasks at hand.

Physical health may also be a factor competing with the caregiving role. As people age, they are more likely to develop chronic illnesses (Verbrugge, 1989) as well as experience general health declines in, for example, vision and hearing (Madden, 1990; Merrill & Verbrugge, 1999). Those with ill health may be unable to physically assist relatives who need to be lifted out of beds or bathtubs, and people with vision problems might have trouble reading labels on medicine bottles. Some individuals who have been carefully managing their diets and exercising regularly may be better able to help with some physical aspects of the caregiving role.

Psychosocial development in middle adulthood has been the focus of considerable research, some of which has been aimed at middle adult caregivers. Individuals in middle adulthood who provide care for a parent may be reciprocating the care their parents originally provided to them. Erikson (1980) termed this impulse to fulfill social responsibilities *generativity*. Peterson (2002) found that women who had more generativity at age 43 perceived less burden in caregiving for their parents 10 years later.

Individuals in middle adulthood are likely to have the largest *convoys* (i.e., circles of close friends and family members; Antonucci, Akiyama, & Merline, 2001), especially women. Consequently, compared with younger and older caregivers, middle adult caregivers should have the most social support available. This may not be true for specific individuals for reasons such as poor health limiting their ability to maintain their social network (Shifren, 1996). A reduction in the number of family and friends that middle adult caregivers have as available resources could also be due to a deliberate reduction in this network by the caregiver: As people get older, they may be more selective about the family and friends they choose to have around them (Carstensen, Isaacowitz, & Charles, 1999).

In keeping with the life span development theory that development is dependent on context, it is important to discuss ethnic and cultural differences in caregiving samples. Many studies of the caregiving experience do take these differences into account. For example, research on middle adult caregivers has shown that there may be ethnic and cultural differences in the amount of social support available to caregivers. White-Means and Rubin (2003) used the 2000 Health and Retirement Study database (National Institute on Aging, 2007) to study caregivers from different ethnic backgrounds. African American caregivers in middle adulthood were less likely to be married, were less educated, had lower income, had more children, and were more likely to provide assistance with ADLs than Caucasian American caregivers. African American mothers and fathers needed more assistance with ADLs than Caucasian mothers and fathers and were less able to be left alone for more than 1 hour. White-Means and Rubin found that African American families with more children available to provide help actually received less help from their children with finances and reminders about medication than African American caregivers from smaller families. However, even African American caregivers from large families received more support than caregivers in Caucasian American families.

Research on middle adult caregivers is vast, and results from a number of these studies are summarized in chapter 5 in this volume, which focuses on women in their 40s to early 60s who are caregiving for a parent or adult relative while raising their children. The authors review the studies they have conducted on women who are middle adult caregivers. They summarize the results of their programmatic research on theoretical perspectives about women's multiple roles, including two hypotheses—the competing demands hypothesis and the expansion hypothesis. They describe important changes in history and context that have affected women in midlife and the multiple roles of women, including that of mother, wife, and employee. They provide evidence that helping women gain meaning and purpose from their multiple roles improves their psychological well-being.

OLDER ADULT CAREGIVERS AND LIFE SPAN DEVELOPMENT

In individuals 65 and older physical and cognitive changes take place that could affect their ability to provide care for aging parents and other older adult relatives. Unfortunately, as people live longer, their risk for illness and disability increases (Verbrugge, 1989). For example, some older adults may be contending with bone loss (*osteoporosis*) or visual loss resulting from cataracts (National Center for Health Statistics, 2007). Bone loss can be detrimental to health (National Center for Health Statistics, 2007), and visual loss can interfere with daily activities such as reading and can increase the likelihood of falls (Ivers, Cumming, Mitchell, & Attebo, 1998). High-frequency hearing loss can interfere with the perception of speech (Mulrow et al., 1990). Obviously, these kinds of changes in physical development can affect a caregiver's ability to read or hear medical instructions for a care recipient as well as impede social interactions.

The average person generally assumes that cognitive changes are inevitable with increasing age. However, unless some form of dementia strikes, most older adults do not show much in the way of cognitive losses until they reach their 70s, and performance does not decline below the average cognitive level of young adults until individuals reach their 80s (Schaie, 1996). The research on cognition and aging is vast and varied. There is evidence for significant declines in performance on some cognitive tasks but stability in others. Declines in the ability to perform certain cognitive tasks may affect the older adult caregiver's ability to perform the caregiving role. Effective caregiving means being able to perform multiple tasks such as dressing and bathing a care recipient while at the same time remembering to take care of other necessities (e.g., administering correct medications and preparing the correct foods). Working memory involves the ability to hold and manipulate information simultaneously (Park et al., 2003). It is important to understand how changes in working memory can affect the caregiver. For example, a caregiver must remember not only the dosage of a medication to give to a care recipient but the side effects of the medication as well.

Older adults do not perform as well as younger adults on most working memory tasks (Park et al., 2003). However, there is some evidence for less decline in working memory tasks involving emotional material rather than visual information (Mikels, Larkin, Lorenz-Reuter, & Carstensen, 2005). Once significant declines in working memory performance are present, the ability to perform multiple tasks necessary for caregiving may be diminished. From a neurological point of view, older adults show different neural activation patterns than younger adults for the same working memory tasks (Park et al., 2003).

Other cognitive changes are important. Older adults do not perform as well as younger adults on tasks of episodic memory (e.g., recall, source memory), but the two groups show little age difference for semantic memory tasks (e.g., lexical decisions, semantic priming; Zacks, Hasher, & Li, 2000). It is important to note that the procedural memory and world knowledge of adults appear to remain stable as they age (Schaie, 2005). Therefore, unless some form of dementia strikes an older adult caregiver, he or she is likely to be able to remember how to do the tasks necessary for caregiving.

Psychosocial development in older adulthood involves important changes. As with younger caregivers, the ability to maintain a social network is important for older adult caregivers' well-being and physical health. Kiecolt-Glaser, Dura, Speicher, Trask, and Glaser (1991) studied spouse caregivers of dementia patients with low amounts of social support during the initial assessment and found poorer immune function 1 year later. Even more so than in middle adulthood, as people age, they appear to become more selective about the individuals in their social network (Carstensen et al., 1999). Older adults who are ill may choose to associate only with individuals who help them maintain better well-being and physical health (Shifren, 1996).

In terms of the caregiving role itself, the social support provided by caregivers to care recipients is important. Social support, whether for assistance because of the care recipient's level of pain (Martire et al., 2006; Parris Stephens, Martire, Cremeans-Smith, Druley, & Wojno, 2006) or because of dementia-related needs (Roth, Mittelman, Clay, Madan, & Haley, 2005), is an important aspect of the caregiver–care recipient relationship. For example, the quality of social support can affect the level of communication about pain in osteoarthritis patients, and this can affect the well-being of the caregiver and the care recipient. Martire et al. (2006) found that spouses who accurately perceive the amount of pain experienced by a partner with osteoarthritis were able to manage the caregiving role with less irritation. In fact, perceptions of caregivers on the level of functioning of care recipients may be crucial to the ability to perform the caregiving role. Shaver and Allan (2004) found that there was less agreement between care receiver and caregiver on the presence of disability for men than for women, especially for those care receivers who were 75 to 84 years old. Overall, care receivers reported higher functioning than the caregivers attributed to them.

As mentioned earlier, there has been extensive research on caregiving in older adult samples, with ethnicity and culture being important variables. Weiss, González, Kabeto, and Langa (2005) used the 1993 Asset and Health Dynamics (AHEAD) study (Soldo, Hurd, Rodgers, & Wallace, 1997) with 7,443 individuals to examine differences in the amount of informal care received by non-Hispanic Caucasian Americans, African Americans, and Hispanic Americans in a nationally representative probability sample of community dwellers aged 70 and older. They found that more elderly Hispanic Americans received informal care (44.3%) than either elderly African Americans (33.9%) or elderly non-Hispanic Caucasian Americans (24.6%). Weiss et al. argued that cultural values may have played a role in this difference. Roff et al. (2004) found that African American caregivers scored lower on anxiety and were less bothered by care recipients' behavior than Caucasian American caregivers. Mak (2005) found that African American caregivers better controlled more troublesome behaviors of the care recipients than Caucasian American caregivers.

One area that has only recently received attention is that of grandparent caregivers. Although even young adults may become grandparents, the majority of grandparents are in middle and older adulthood. Though grandparenthood can begin as early as age 30, the average age to begin grandparenthood is about 48 years old (Davies & Williams, 2002). There are about 30% of grandparent caregivers age 60 and older. Because people now live longer than ever before, individuals can expect to be grandparent caregivers for at least several decades if they are healthy enough to continue the role. Someone may become a grandparent caregiver to a grandchild for a variety of reasons—for example, if the child's parent dies, is incarcerated, becomes addicted to drugs, or has mental health problems (Allen, Philliber, Herrling, & Kuperminc, 1997). Regardless of the reason, today in the United States more than 2.4 million grandparents provide basic caregiving for grandchildren who live with them (Davies & Williams, 2002). More than 50% of these families are members of minority groups, and 19% of grandparent caregivers have household incomes at the poverty level (U.S. Census Bureau, 2003).

Chapter 6 of this volume provides a strong argument to support the use of life span development principles in grandparent caregiver research. The authors summarize their studies on grandparent caregivers and review additional research on grandparent caregivers. They discuss how the historical and contextual aspects of development have led to increasing numbers of grandparent caregivers, and they present information on the multidimensional aspects of being grandparent caregivers. They also discuss factors that have been studied within the *stress and coping model framework* (a cognitive view of how people evaluate events; see Lazarus & Folkman, 1984) for caregiving research, and then they tie that back into the larger life span development perspective about caregivers. Patrick and Goedereis provide descriptions of research on grandparent caregivers involving the stress and coping model framework, and they describe how the model has been modified for use with this group. Finally, they present recent data on an emerging adult sample to address a newer area of research related to grandparent caregivers: long-term effects of living with and being raised by grandparents. Specifically, they assess emerging adults' attitudes and views toward grandparent caregiving, including whether coresidence and child rearing by grandparents led to emerging adults being more supportive of coresiding with their own children and parents once they reach middle adulthood.

A CLOSING NOTE

My own research on the effects of early caregiving on adult development and aging involves the principles of life span development, and it was inspired by my own life. Perhaps my own experiences as a caregiver can help you think about caregiving from a life span perspective. I was 14 years old when my mother had a major heart attack that caused severe damage to her heart. Four more heart attacks followed when I was 18; 21; 30; and, most recently, 35 years old. I became a mother during my most recent episode of caregiving for my mom. I helped my mother with everything—bathing and dressing, medications, surgical bandage changes, and housework—for as long as she needed it. Each time I experienced life as a caregiver, my developmental stage affected my caregiving role, and my caregiving role affected my development in turn.

At the time I write this chapter, my mother is still alive, and although ill, she provides lots of love and care for my two young children at least once a week. Helping her to be here to share in the lives of her grandchildren is a very positive reward for my help to her. I am now in middle adulthood and do not know what other caregiving roles I will take on. I do know that my prior experiences have affected and will continue to affect my mind and my behaviors over time.

My thanks go out to the reviewers for this book who spent considerable time and effort going through each chapter and providing much-needed constructive criticisms of the book. The efforts were greatly appreciated, and the revised chapters are much stronger because of the reviewers' comments. I am especially grateful for the efforts of the editorial and production staff at the American Psychological Association Books Department who worked diligently with me to improve the flow of information. I am indebted to my colleague, Karen Hooker, who helped me to develop a true passion for research on caregiving and the importance of the life span development perspective when I was her dissertation student at Syracuse University. May I one day be as fine a researcher (and writer) as she. I am honored to have the privilege of working with such great researchers to create this book. Thanks to each of you for your excellent and timely work. Last, but certainly not least, I am deeply grateful for the support and patience of my family while my colleagues and I have worked on the chapters in this book. Thanks Bob, Alexander, and Kayla.

REFERENCES

Allen, J. P., Philliber, S., Herrling, S., & Kuperminc, G. P. (1997). Preventing teen pregnancy and academic failure: Experimental evaluation of a developmentally based approach. *Child Development, 64,* 729–742.

Antonucci, T. C., Akiyama, H., & Merline, A. (2001). Dynamics of social relationships in midlife. In M. E. Lachman (Ed.), *Handbook of midlife development* (pp. 571–598). New York: Wiley.

Arnett, J. J. (1998). Learning to stand alone: The contemporary American transition to adulthood in cultural and historical context. *Human Development, 41,* 295–315.

Arnett, J. J. (2000). Emerging adulthood: A theory of development from the late teens through the twenties. *American Psychologist, 55,* 469–480.

Baltes, P. B. (1987). Theoretical propositions of life-span development psychology: On the dynamics between growth and decline. *Developmental Psychology, 23,* 611–626.

Baltes, P. B., Lindenberger, U., & Staudinger, U. M. (1998). Life-span theory in developmental psychology. In R. M. Lerner (Ed.), *Handbook of child psychology: Vol. 1. Theoretical models of human development* (pp. 1029–1143). New York: Wiley.

Baltes, P. B., Staudinger, U. M., & Lindenberger, U. (1999). Lifespan psychology: Theory and application to intellectual functioning. *Annual Review of Psychology, 50,* 471–507.

Basseches, M. (1984). *Dialectical thinking and adult development.* Norwood, NJ: Ablex.

Basseches, M. (1989). Dialectical thinking as an organized whole: Comments on Irwin and Kramer. In M. L. Commons, J. D. Sinnott, F. A. Richards, & C. Armon (Eds.), *Adult development, Vol. 1: Comparisons and applications of developmental models* (pp. 161–178). New York: Praeger.

Beach, D. L. (1997). Family caregiving: The positive impact on adolescent relationships. *The Gerontologist, 37,* 233–238.

Boerner, K., Schulz, R., & Horowitz, A. (2004). Positive aspects of care giving and adaptation to bereavement. *Psychology and Aging, 19,* 668–675.

Bronfenbrenner, U. (1986). Ecology of the family as a context for human development: Research perspectives. *Developmental Psychology, 22,* 723–742.

Burton, L. M., Obeidallah, D. A., & Allison, K. (1996). Ethnographic insights on social context and adolescent development among inner-city African American teens. In R. Jessor, A. Colby, & R. A. Shweder (Eds.), *Ethnography and human development: Context and meaning in social inquiry* (pp. 375–415). Chicago: University of Chicago Press.

Carstensen, L. L., Isaacowitz, D. M., & Charles, S. T. (1999). Taking time seriously: A theory of socioemotional selectivity. *American Psychologist, 54,* 165–181.

Danielsen, L. M., Lorem, A. E., & Kroger, J. (2000). The impact of social context on the identity-formation process of Norwegian late adolescents. *Youth and Society, 31,* 332–363.

Davies, C., & Williams, D. (2002). *The grandparent study 2002 report.* Retrieved April 9, 2008, from http://assets.aarp.org/rgcenter/general/gp_2002.pdf

Dearden, C., & Becker, S. (1999). The experiences of young carers in the UK: The mental health issues. *Mental Health Care, 2,* 273–276.

Dellmann-Jenkins, M., Blankemeyer, M., & Pinkard, O. (2001). Incorporating the elder caregiving role into the developmental tasks of young adulthood. *Journal of Aging and Human Development, 52,* 1–18.

Dellmann-Jenkins, M., & Brittain, L. (2003). Young adults' attitudes toward filial responsibility and actual assistance to elderly family members. *Journal of Applied Gerontology, 22,* 214–229.

Elder, G. H., Jr. (1974). *Children of the Great Depression: Social change in life experience.* Chicago: University of Chicago Press.

Elder, G. H., Jr., George, L. K., & Shanahan, M. J. (1996). Psychosocial stress over the life course. In H. B. Kaplan's *Psychosocial stress: Perspectives on structure, theory, life-course, and methods* (pp. 247–292). San Diego, CA: Academic Press.

Erikson. E. H. (1963). *Childhood and society.* New York: Norton.

Erikson, E. H. (1968). *Identity: Youth and crisis.* New York: Norton.

Erikson, E. H. (1980). *Identity and the life cycle.* New York: Norton.

Galotti, K. M., Komatsu, L. K., & Voelz, J. (1997). Children's differential performance on deductive and inductive syllogisms. *Developmental Psychology, 33,* 70–78.

Garmezy, N. (1993). Children in poverty: Resilience despite risk. *Psychiatry, 56,* 127–136.

Gates, M. F., & Lackey, N. R. (1998). Youngsters caring for adults with cancer. *Image: Journal of Nursing Scholarship, 30,* 11–15.

Goldscheider, F., & Goldscheider, C. (1994). Leaving and returning home in 20th century America. *Population Bulletin, 48,* 1–35.

Greene, A. L., Wheatley, S. M., & Aldava, J. F., IV. (1992). Stages on life's way: Adolescents' implicit theories of the lifecourse. *Journal of Adolescent Research, 7,* 364–381.

Haley, W. E. (2003). The costs of family care giving: Implications for geriatric oncology. *Critical Reviews in Oncology/Hematology, 48,* 151–159.

Harter, S. (1990). Causes, correlates, and the functional role of global self-worth: A life-span perspective. In J. Kolligan & R. Sternberg (Eds.), *Competence considered: Perceptions of competence and incompetence across the lifespan* (pp. 67–97). New Haven, CT: Yale University Press.

Hooker, K. (1992). Possible selves and perceived health in older adults and college students. *Journal of Gerontology, 47,* P85–P95.

Hooker, K., Frazier, L. D., & Monahan, D. J. (1994). Personality and coping among caregivers of spouses with dementia. *The Gerontologist, 34,* 386–392.

Hooker, K., Manoogian-O'Dell, M., Monahan, D. J., Frazier, L. D., & Shifren, K. (2000). Does type of disease matter? Gender differences among Alzheimer's and Parkinson's disease spouse caregivers. *The Gerontologist, 40,* 568–573.

Hooker, K., Monahan, D. J., Bowman, S. R., Frazier, L. D., & Shifren, K. (1998). Personality counts for a lot: Predictors of mental and physical health of spouse caregivers in two disease groups. *Journal of Gerontology: Psychological Sciences: 53B,* P73–P85.

Hunt, G., Levine, C., & Naiditch, L. (2005). *Young caregivers in the U.S.: Findings from a national survey.* Retrieved March 19, 2008, from http://www.uhfnyc.org/usr_doc/Young_Caregivers_Study_083105.pdf

Ivers, R. O., Cumming, R. G., Mitchell, P., & Attebo, K. (1998). Visual impairment and falls in older adults: The Blue Mountains Eye Study. *Journal of the American Geriatric Society, 46,* 58–64.

Jastrzembski, T. S., Charness, N., & Vasyukova, C. (2006). Expertise and age effects on knowledge activation in chess. *Psychology and Aging, 21,* 401–405.

Kerpelman, J. L., Shoffner, M. F., & Ross-Griffin, S. (2002). African American mothers' and daughters' beliefs about possible selves and their strategies for reaching the adolescents' future academic and career goals. *Journal of Youth and Adolescence, 31,* 289–303.

Kiecolt-Glaser, J. K., Dura, J. R., Speicher, C. E., Trask, O. J., & Glaser, R. (1991). Spousal caregivers of dementia victims: Longitudinal changes in immunity and health. *Psychosomatic Medicine, 53,* 345–362.

Labouvie-Vief, G. (1998). Cognitive–emotional integration in adulthood. In K. W. Schaie & M. P. Lawton (Eds.), *Annual review of gerontology and geriatrics: Vol. 17. Focus on emotion and adult development.* (pp. 206–237). New York: Springer Publishing Company.

Lachman, M. E. (2004). Development in midlife. *Annual Review of Psychology, 55,* 305–331.

Lachman, M. E., & James, J. B. (1997). Charting the course of midlife development: An overview. In M. E. Lachman & J. B. James (Eds.), *Multi-*

ple paths of midlife development (pp. 1–17). Chicago: University of Chicago Press.

Lackey, N. R., & Gates, M. F. (1997). Combining the analyses of three data sets in studying young caregivers. *Journal of Advanced Nursing, 26,* 664–671.

Lackey, N. R., & Gates, M. F. (2001). Adults' recollection of their experiences as young caregivers of family members with chronic physical illnesses. *Journal of Advanced Nursing, 34,* 320–328.

Lazarus, R. S., & Folkman, S. (1984). *Stress, appraisal, and coping.* New York: Springer Publishing Company.

Levine, C., Hunt, G. G., Halper, D., Hart, A. Y., Lautz, J., & Gould, D. A. (2005). Young adults caregivers: A first look at an unstudied population. *American Journal of Public Health, 95,* 2071–2075.

Madan-Swain, A., Brown, R. T., & Foster, M.A. (2000). Identity in adolescent survivors of childhood cancer. *Journal of Pediatric Psychology, 25,* 105–115.

Madden, D. J. (1990). Adult age differences in the time course of visual attention. *Journal of Gerontology: Psychological Sciences, 45,* P9–P16.

Mak, W. W. (2005). Integrative model of caregiving: How macro and micro factors affect caregivers of adults with severe and persistent mental illness. *American Journal of Orthopsychiatry, 75,* 40–53.

Martire, L. M., Keefe, F. J., Schulz, R., Ready, R., Beach, S. R., Rudy, T. E., & Starz, T. W. (2006). Older spouses' perceptions of partners' chronic arthritis pain: Implications for spousal responses, support provision, and care giving experiences. *Psychology and Aging, 21,* 222–230.

Masten, A. S., & Coatsworth, J. D. (1998). The development of competence in favorable and unfavorable environments: Lessons from research on successful children. *American Psychologist, 53,* 205–220.

Masten, A. A., Coatsworth, J. D., Neemann, J., Gest, S. D., Tellegen, A., & Garmezy, N. (1995). The structure and coherence of competence from childhood through adolescence. *Child Development, 66,* 1635–1659.

Masten, A. S., Hubbard, J. J., Gest, S. D., Tellegen, A., Garmezy, N., & Ramirez, N. (1999). Competence in the context of adversity: Pathways to resilience and maladaptation from childhood to late adolescence. *Developmental Psychopathology, 11,* 143–169.

Merrill, S. S., & Verbrugge, L. M. (1999). Health and disease in midlife. In S. L. Willis & J. D. Reid (Eds.), *Life in the middle: Psychological and social development in middle age* (pp. 78–103). San Diego, CA: Academic Press.

Mikels, J. A., Larkin, G. R., Lorenz-Reuter, P.A., & Carstensen, L. L. (2005). Divergent trajectories in the aging mind: Changes in working memory for affective versus visual information with age. *Psychology and Aging, 20,* 542–553.

Mulrow, C. D., Aguilar, C., Endicott, J. E., Tuley, M. R., Velez, R., Charlip, W. S., et al. (1990). Quality of life changes and hearing impairment: A randomized trial. *Annals of Internal Medicine, 113,* 188–194.

National Alliance for Caregiving & the American Association of Retired Persons. (2004). *Caregiving in the U.S.* Washington, DC: Author.

National Center for Health Statistics. (2007). *Older persons' health.* Retrieved March 18, 2008, from http://www.cdc.gov/nchs/fastats/older_americans.htm

National Institute on Aging. (2007). *Growing older in America: The Health and Retirement Study.* Retrieved April 14, 2008, from http://www.nia.nih.gov/ResearchInformation/extramuralPrograms/BehavioralandSocialResearch/HRS.htm

Nolen-Hoeksema, S., & Ahrens, C. (2002). Age differences and similarities in the correlates of depressive symptoms. *Psychology and Aging, 17,* 116–124.

Papalia, D. E., Olds, S. W., & Feldman, R. D. (2007). *Human development* (10th ed.). New York: McGraw-Hill.

Park, D. C., Welsh, R. C., Marshuetz, C., Gutchess, A. H., Mikels, J., Polk, T. A., et al. (2003). Working memory for complex scenes: Age differences in frontal and hippocampus activations. *Journal of Cognitive Neuroscience, 15,* 1122–1134.

Parris Stephens, M. A., Martire, L. M., Cremeans-Smith, J. K., Druley, J. A., & Wojno, W. C. (2006). Older women with osteoarthritis and their care giving husbands: Effects of pain and pain expression on husbands' well-being and support. *Rehabilitation Psychology, 51,* 3–12.

Peterson, B. E. (2002). Longitudinal analysis of midlife generativity, intergenerational roles, and care giving. *Psychology and Aging, 17,* 161–168.

Piaget, J., & Inhelder, B. (1967). *The child's conception of space.* New York: Norton.

Pinquart, M., & Sörensen, S. (2003). Associations of stressors and uplifts of care giving with caregiver burden and depressive mood: A meta-analysis. *The Journals of Gerontology Series B: Psychological Sciences and Social Sciences, 58B,* 112–129.

Pinquart, M., & Sörensen, S. (2005). Ethnic differences in stressors, resources, and psychological outcomes of family care giving: A meta-analysis. *The Gerontologist, 45,* 90–116.

Robertson, S. M., Zarit, S. H., Duncan, L. G., Rovine, M. J., & Femia, E. E. (2007). Family caregivers' patterns of positive and negative affect. *Family Relations, 56,* 12–23.

Roff, L. L., Burgio, L. D., Gitlin, L., Nichols, L., Chaplin, W , & Hardin, M. (2004). Positive aspects of Alzheimer's care giving: The role of race. *Journals of Gerontology Series B: Psychological Sciences and Social Sciences, 59B,* P185–P190.

Roth, D. L., Mittelman, M. S., Clay, O. J., Madan, A., & Haley, W. E. (2005). Changes in social support as mediators of the impact of a psychosocial intervention for spouse caregivers of persons with Alzheimer's disease. *Psychology and Aging, 20,* 634–644.

Schaie, K. W. (1996). Intellectual development in adulthood. In J. E. Birren & K. W. Schaie (Eds.), *Handbook of the psychology of aging* (4th ed., pp. 266–286). San Diego, CA: Academic Press.

Schaie, K. W. (2005). *Developmental influences on adult intelligence: The Seattle Longitudinal Study.* New York: Oxford University Press.

Shaver, J. C., & Allan, D. E. (2004). Care-receiver and caregiver assessment of functioning: Are there gender differences? *Canadian Journal of Aging, 24,* 139–150.

Shifren, K. (1996). Individual differences in the perception of optimism and disease severity: A 70 day study among individuals with Parkinson's disease. *Journal of Behavioral Medicine, 19,* 241–271.

Shifren, K. (2008). *Early caregiving: Perceived parental relations and current health and social support.* Manuscript under review.

Shifren, K., Furnham, A., & Bauserman, R. L. (1998). Instrumental and expressive traits and eating attitudes: A replication across American and British students. *Personality and Individual Differences, 25,* 1–17.

Shifren, K., Furnham, A., & Bauserman, R. L. (2003). Emerging adulthood in American and British samples: Individuals' personality and health risk behaviors. *Journal of Adult Development, 10,* 75–88.

Shifren, K., & Hooker, K. (1995). Stability and change in optimism; A study among spouse caregivers. *Experimental Aging Research, 21,* 59–76.

Shifren, K., & Kachorek, L. V. (2003). Does early care giving matter? The effects on young caregivers' adult mental health. *International Journal of Behavioral Development, 27,* 338–346.

Sinnott, J. D. (1998*). The development of logic in adulthood: Postformal thought and its applications.* New York: Plenum Press.

Siskowski, C. T. (2006). Young caregivers: Effect of family health situations on school performance. *Journal of School Nursing, 22,* 163–169.

Soederberg Miller, L. M., & Lachman, M. E. (2000). Cognitive performance and the role of control beliefs in midlife. *Aging, Neuropsychology, and Cognition, 7,* 69–85.

Smith, T. W., & Rhodewalt, F. (1986). On states, traits, and processes: A transactional alternative to the individual difference assumptions in Type A behavior and physiological reactivity. *Journal of Research in Personality, 20,* 229–251.

Soldo, B. J., Hurd, M. D., Rodgers, W. L., & Wallace, R. B. (1997). Asset and health dynamics among the oldest old: An overview of the AHEAD study. *The Journal of Gerontology: Series B, 52B,* 1–20.

Stein, C. H., Wemmerus, V.A., Ward, M., Gaines, M. E., Freeberg, A. L., & Jewell, T. C. (1998). "Because they're my parents": An intergenerational study of felt obligation and parental care giving. *Journal of Marriage and Family, 60*, 611–622.

Tiet, Q. Q., Bird, H. R., Davies, M., Hoven, C., Cohen, P., Jensen, P. S., & Goodman, S. (1998). Adverse life events and resilience. *Journal of the American Academy of Child and Adolescent Psychiatry, 37*, 1191–2000.

U.S. Census Bureau. (2003, October). *Grandparents living with grandchildren: 2000. Census 2000 brief.* Retrieved April 14, 2008, from http://www.census.gov/prod/2003pubs/c2kbr-31.pdf

Verbrugge, L. M. (1989). The twain meet: Empirical explanations of sex differences in health and mortality. *Journal of Health and Social Behavior, 30*, 282–304.

Vitaliano, P. P., Zhang, J., & Scanlan, J. M. (2003). Is care giving hazardous to one's physical health? A meta-analysis. *Psychological Bulletin, 129*, 946–972.

Weiss, C. O., González, H. M., Kabeto, M. U., & Langa, K. M. (2005). Differences in amount of informal care received by non-Hispanic Whites and Latinos in a nationally representative sample of older Americans. *Journal of the American Geriatrics Society, 53*, 146–151.

White-Means, S. J., & Rubin, R. M. (2003). Racial differences in dilemmas of the "sandwich generation". *Consumer Interests Annual, 49*, 1–4.

Willis, S. L., & Schaie, K. W. (1999). Intellectual functioning in midlife. In S. L. Willis & J. D. Reid (Eds.), *Life in the middle: Psychological and social development in middle age* (pp. 233–247). Boston: Academic Press.

Yee, J. L., & Schulz, R. (2000). Gender differences in psychiatric morbidity among family caregivers: A review and analysis. *The Gerontologist, 40*, 147–164.

Yoder, A. E. (2000). Barriers to ego identity status formation: A contextual qualification of Marcia's identity status. *Journal of Adolescence, 23*, 95–107.

Zacks, R. T., Hasher, L., & Li, K. Z. H. (2000). Human memory. In T. A. Salthouse & F. I. M. Craik (Eds.), *Handbook of aging and cognition* (2nd ed., pp. 293–357). Mahwah, NJ: Erlbaum.

1

Children as Caregivers to Their Ill Parents With AIDS

Laurie J. Bauman, Ellen Johnson Silver,
Rebecca Berman, and Ivy Gamble

Within the life span development framework, one key principle is that development is dependent on history (Baltes, Lindenberger, & Staudinger, 1998). An important aspect of the history of the United States was the presence of HIV/AIDS in the 1980s and the rapid increase in this life-threatening disease after its arrival (Papalia, Olds, & Feldman, 2007). HIV/AIDS has changed the meaning of childhood for children in many ways, but one of the least recognized is the hidden burden healthy children bear as caregivers to ill parents with HIV/AIDS. This is particularly evident when parental HIV/AIDS forces changes in usual family roles to accommodate an ill mother's need for care (Cates, Graham, Boeglin, & Tiekler, 1990; C. Levine, 1990, 1995). The purpose of this chapter is to report data from a study on children of mothers with and without HIV/AIDS in New York City. Our study examined how much responsibility the children assumed for caregiving and household chores when their mothers had HIV/AIDS. We also looked at whether certain children, such as older children or daughters, were more likely to take on these responsibilities and what effects (both negative and positive) this had on the children. It may seem odd to consider young children as caregivers, but it is

Portions of this chapter were presented in a poster session at the National Institute of Mental Health Conference on the Role of Families in Preventing and Adapting to HIV/AIDS, Washington, DC, July 2003. We are grateful to the Ittleson Foundation and to the National Institute of Mental Health (Grant 5R01MH55794) for funding this research and to Willo Pequegnat for her support, dedication, and leadership in research on the role of families in adapting to HIV/AIDS. We thank Michele J. Siegel for conducting part of the analysis, Marni Loiacono for assistance with manuscript preparation, and the families who so generously gave their time to participate.

not uncommon to find children fulfilling roles and responsibilities usually defined as appropriate for adults. Therefore, it is most fitting to begin this book on the developmental implications of the role of caregiver with the youngest caregivers.

Developmentally, the role of caregiver is unexpected in childhood. Children become caregivers when situations force them to, when their parents are not well enough to parent. Children may become the de facto heads of their households, assuming adult responsibilities, experiencing adult anxieties, and making adult decisions. The risk developmentally is that children may become *parentified*, that is, they take on responsibilities more appropriately handled by adults, such as providing health and personal care or emotional support, caring for siblings, and maintaining the household. Parentification occurs when older children seek outside paid employment to support their family or when they act as parents to their younger siblings—children raising children. It also occurs when children care for a parent who is seriously ill and may be dying. Some children are the main caregivers for their ill parents, washing and feeding a bedridden mother or father, administering medication, or acting as a confidant, although many others share these responsibilities with an adult or a sibling. Little is known about the extent to which children provide health and personal care to ill parents; how often they assume household responsibilities for cooking, marketing, and maintenance; and how often they provide care to siblings. In addition, little is known about the emotional or developmental consequences for children of taking on this type of responsibility. It also is not known how often children with ill parents miss school or other critical activities because of their responsibilities or because they lack necessary funds or other resources.

A series of surveys in Great Britain (Becker, October 2003–April 2004; Becker & Dearden, October 2004–April 2005) has provided some of the most comprehensive data to date on child caregivers. According to data from the 2001 U.K. census, there were 175,000 young caregivers under age 18, of whom 13,000 looked after or provided some type of unpaid service to a sick, disabled, or elderly person more than 50 hours per week, but little else was known about these young people (Becker, October 2003–April

2004). However, in 2003, a national survey was conducted that gathered data on 6,178 young caregivers under age 18 who were supported by 87 support services projects across the United Kingdom. This was the third of three national surveys (others were done in 1995 and 1997). The data on the young caregivers were provided by the projects that responded. Two thirds of these children cared for a parent. Their average age of 12 hid the fact that 29% were 5 to 10 years of age. More than one half lived in single-parent families, suggesting that the absence of a second parent increases the likelihood of a child taking on the caregiving role. Their reported duties included household chores (cooking, cleaning, etc.) and management (e.g., bill paying), emotional support, intimate care (washing, dressing, toileting), and child care. Increased age was associated with increased responsibility. Almost one half spent about 10 hours per week in caregiving, but one third provided care between 11 and 20 hours per week and another 18% did so for more than 20 hours per week. Caregiving was a long-term commitment for many, lasting at least 3 years for 2 out of 3 children. Responsibilities were related to a wide range of consequences: friendship difficulties, limited time for social or leisure activities, difficult or problematic transition into adulthood, missed school, limited time for schoolwork, and educational problems.

Robson (2000, 2004), who conducted in-depth qualitative interviews with child caregivers aged 15 to 17 years in Zimbabwe, found that most provided intimate personal care as well as treatment-related and household duties. All recipients required full-time care and help with daily living. Girls were usually responsible for the care of an ill person. Girls often were taken out of school for this duty, whereas boys more commonly continued their education. Children seem to become caregivers on the basis of degree of illness, availability of support services, poverty, family structure, coresidence, gender, age, educational level, and income-earning ability. Thomas et al. (2003) interviewed 17 young caregivers aged 9 to 18 years and conducted focus groups with 38 more. Half were struggling in school and many had trouble obtaining health services for themselves and felt their knowledge about their parent's illness often went ignored. Young caregivers in this study reported problems with peers, depression, worry, stress, and fear. Most reported no outside recognition; at times, schools did not believe or understand the situation, but at other times, the children felt schools tried too hard and were overly intrusive when they kept asking them questions about how they were doing at home. Caregivers also reported positive aspects, including obtaining useful experience, being better prepared to live independently, and placing a high value on family life. Many reported that they did not want to be "rescued" from their roles or separated from their families.

A recent national survey of 213 U.S. child caregivers aged 8 to 18 included a comparison group of 250 noncaregivers (Hunt, Levine, & Naiditch, 2005). The authors estimated that there are 1.3 million to 1.4 million child caregivers in the United States in this age range and about one third are 11 years old or younger. About one half of the children studied were boys, and 72% were caring for a parent or grandparent. Most children did not provide care on their own; 3 out of 4 child caregivers had help. Duties included helping with activities of daily living (e.g., feeding, washing, dressing, using the bathroom), helping with medications, making appointments for care, paying bills or doing other household paperwork, grocery shopping, preparing meals, and helping the care recipient get around in the community. Some also cared for siblings. Overall, 15% of child caregivers said that the care recipients talked about things that they did not discuss with others. Girls (21%) were twice as likely as boys (10%) to say that the care recipient confided in them. Child caregivers in this study reported both positive and negative aspects of caregiving. Problems included anxiety and depression and having less time for themselves. Positives included feeling appreciated for the help they gave, that they had productive days, and that adults listened to them. Children who provided care did not have lower self-esteem or higher sadness or loneliness than children who did not.

A study of 11,029 public school students in Grades 6 through 12 in Palm Beach, Florida (Siskowski, 2004), found that 56% contributed to the care of a person with special medical needs. Children reported that caregiving affected their academic performance (67.3%), interfered with learning (38.5%), or interrupted their thinking or time studying (24.2%). In addition, 17.1% said that they did not complete homework assignments, and 13.2% said that they missed school or after school activities.

Parentification in child caregivers can include *role reversal*, where a child acts as if he or she were the parent. Some children, particularly girls, become confidants to their ill parents and provide emotional support when their parents are depressed or afraid. Bauman, Phuong, Silver, and Berman (2001) found that daughters who provided emotional support to an ill mother with AIDS had significantly more self-reported symptoms of depression than those who did not provide this type of support, but their ill parents are unaware of the emotional cost to their daughters. In a study of adolescent children of women with HIV/AIDS, parentification was found to be more common among girls and when the parent used drugs and was more ill, and it was associated with increased internalizing symptoms (depression, anxiety, somaticization) and some externalizing problem behaviors (conduct problems, sexual behavior, alcohol, and marijuana use) in these adolescents (Stein, Riedel, & Rotheram-Borus, 1999). However, a recent study of youth ages 9 to 16 years, some of whom were affected by maternal HIV infection, indicated that parentification involving increased emotional closeness rather than solely household maintenance tasks is associated with lower rates of self-reported depressive symptoms (Tompkins, 2007). Inhibited or delayed development, depression, guilt, and low self-esteem are all possible outcomes when children take on the parenting role (Barnett & Parker, 1998; Wallace, 1996).

This may be related in some respects to the important developmental changes that are taking place in this life stage. According to Eccles (1999), children's development from middle childhood to adolescence is "driven by basic psychological needs to achieve competence, autonomy, and relatedness" (p. 31). The period beginning in middle childhood is particularly critical to developing one's self-identity and individuality, and a child's ability to build healthy self-esteem is highly dependent on his or her being able to competently manage life's successes and failures (Eccles, 1999; M. D. Levine, 1999). Children need a balance in handling positive and negative experiences, and parents are typically their most influential role models in learning how to cope with both. If parents are unavailable, children lose an important resource that helps them build these types of skills. Moreover, children, especially adolescents, who fail at adult tasks may lose confidence in themselves, which can lead to reduced motivation to respond to challenging tasks and learning opportunities and to negative behavior such as truancy, dropping out of school, and early sexual activity (Eccles, 1999).

Some have expressed concern that too much household responsibility can interfere with the time that children need for schoolwork and for socializing with peers (Elkind, 2001). In early adolescence, the child often experiences a growing need for autonomy and distance from the family (Eccles, 1999), and there tend to be more conflicts about family responsibilities and chores. However, it can be argued that successful caregiving experiences may add to a child's sense of competence and to increased maturity. It has been suggested that participating in household work also enhances family cohesiveness (Lee, Schneider, & Waite, 2003).

Recently, we conducted a study of children of parents with HIV/AIDS in Mutare, Zimbabwe, and New York City to document the extent to which children take on adult responsibilities when a parent has HIV/AIDS, the kinds of responsibilities these children have, and the psychological status of child caregivers (Bauman, Foster, Silver, Gamble, & Muchaneta, 2006). We interviewed 50 mothers who were ill from HIV/AIDS in both Mutare, Zimbabwe, and New York City and one child of each (ages 8 through 16). We found that the children provided substantial amounts of personal care and took responsibility for cooking, cleaning, shopping, and other household tasks; some were their parents' confidants. The amount of care provided was related to maternal disability but not to child age, gender, or presence of other adults or siblings. Children reported performing more tasks than their mothers reported. Almost one half of New York children and 80% of Mutare children said that they had too much responsibility, and most reported reduced after school and peer activities. Both children and parents felt that children were more capable because of their responsibilities. We also found that depression rates among children in New York (22%) and Mutare (63%) were high, but Mutare children were extremely vulnerable; nearly two thirds had Child Depression Inventory scores in the clinically significant range (12 or higher). However, child caregiving was unrelated to self-rated depression in either group.

Within life span development theory, a key principle is that development is dependent on context. We addressed the issue of context with an important question about whether the level and impact of children's household responsibilities reported by those in the New York group were specific to inner-city families in which a parent had HIV/AIDS. Without normative community data, we were unable to determine whether any reported experiences of premature caregiving in children in the HIV-affected families we studied were unique or whether they reflected the usual roles of children living with single mothers in highly stressed and economically and socially disadvantaged households in New York. To address this, we designed the current study to collect comparison information from mothers and children in similar but unaffected families. This helps us better understand the importance of context in human development, with and without the caregiving role. We asked each mother already in the New York arm of the previous study to nominate a family from the same community who could be invited to participate in the interview. These families had children in the same age range, and their families were likely to have similar characteristics and face the same challenges related to poverty and lack of support services. This allowed us to isolate the effects of HIV status and investigate whether children in affected families were at higher risk for taking on household responsibilities and for increased emotional or behavioral problems.

Thus, the current study focused on children of parents with and without HIV/AIDS in New York, and had the following aims: (a) to document the extent to which children take on adult responsibilities when a parent has HIV/AIDS, including types of caregiving (health-related personal care; household management) and chores such as cleaning, cooking, washing, shopping, and caring for siblings; (b) to describe which children are more likely to assume caregiving responsibilities (e.g., are older children or daughters at greater risk?); and (c) to describe the consequences of filling the caregiving role for children.

METHOD

Sample and Recruitment

Mothers with HIV/AIDS were recruited from participants in Project Care, a National Institute of Mental Health–funded project to provide succession-planning services to mothers ill with HIV/AIDS. Of the

220 mothers originally enrolled in Project Care, 10 mothers had died and 25 had moved out of state, were too ill to participate, or had been lost to follow-up. Of the 185 families remaining, with 250 children ages 8 to 16 years, we randomly selected families to invite into the new study.

After their interviews were completed, each Project Care mother was asked to nominate a family from the same community to serve as the comparison family. Only a few mothers with HIV/AIDS were unable to provide the name of an eligible comparison mother, and interviewers were successful in obtaining agreement from the referred community mothers.

Measures

The maternal interviews were available in both English and Spanish, and all children were interviewed in English. Whenever possible, we used existing measures that were valid and reliable in interviewing mothers and children, although for this study we developed new measures to describe the child's household responsibilities.

Data collected from the mother included background, family structure, and health status and functional limitations. Questions on household responsibilities included items about personal assistive care needed, how often care was needed and who provided it, the child's routine chores and number of hours per day spent on these chores, and who usually was responsible for other household responsibilities. For tasks that were usually done by the mother, we asked who would do them if she were sick.

Mother's mental health was measured using the Psychiatric Symptom Index (PSI; Ilfeld, 1976), a 29-item self-report scale with good psychometric properties. The PSI measures the intensity of symptoms of depression, anxiety, anger, and cognitive disturbance over the past 2 weeks using a 4-point scale (*never* to *very often*). PSI total and subscale scores have a possible range from 0 to 100 for each scale, and total scores of 20 or above are considered to reflect high levels of psychiatric symptoms (Ilfeld, 1976).

Mothers reported on child mental health using the Child Behavior Checklist (CBCL; Achenbach, 1991a), a parent-report measure of 118 behavioral problems that has a total score as well as internalizing and externalizing subscales and nine symptom subscales. We used the recommended *t*-score transformations of the raw behavior scores, which adjust for age and sex differences in behavior found in normative samples. A *t* score greater than 63 computed for the total score (the highest 10th percentile) or a score above the 97th percentile on any individual subscale indicates clinically meaningful symptoms (Achenbach, 1991a).

In the children's interview we asked about their health, their chores and responsibilities around the house, who took care of their mother when she was not well, who usually took care of household chores, and how things changed when their mother was ill. All children completed the 27-item Children's Depression Inventory (CDI; Kovacs, 1985, 1992). Cronbach's alpha has ranged from .71 to .87 in different studies, and reliability has been demonstrated (Smucker, Craighead, Craighead, & Green, 1986). A CDI score of 12 or higher has been used as the cutoff point to indicate a clinically significant level of symptoms (Barreto & McManus, 1997; Kovacs, 1992).

We also collected data from older children aged 11 to 17 on a different self-report tool, the Youth Self-Report (YSR; Achenbach, 1991b). The YSR is a broad-band measure of symptoms and includes both internalizing symptoms (depression, anxiety, and withdrawal) and externalizing symptoms (conduct problems, oppositional defiant) as well as a total score. YSR items are similar to those in the CBCL, the parent report of behavior described above. As with the CBCL, we used *t*-score transformations of the raw scores and the same recommended clinical cutoff points to indicate likely psychopathology.

Children and mothers reported on the parent–child relationship using different measures. Mothers completed the 44-item form of the Conflict Behavior Questionnaire (CBQ; Prinz, Foster, Kent, & O'Leary, 1979; Robin & Foster, 1989), a measure of negative communication and conflict that the parent–child dyad experiences. It has also been called the Interaction Behavior Questionnaire (Prinz et al., 1979). Parents rate their interactions with their child during the previous 2 weeks in a yes–no or true–false format; two scores are generated, an appraisal of the child and an appraisal of the dyad. Internal consistencies are .88 for the mother's appraisal of the child and .90 for the mother's appraisal of the dyad (Prinz et al., 1979).

The children completed a revised version of the Inventory of Parent and Peer Attachment (IPPA; Armsden & Greenberg, 1987). We used 28 items from the scale that evaluated positive and negative aspects of the parent relationship and the degree to which the mother serves as a source of psychological security. The IPPA was originally designed and validated for older adolescents (16 to 20 years), but its dimensions of trust (degree of mutual understanding and respect), communication (extent and quality), and alienation (feelings of anger and isolation) appeared to be developmentally appropriate for the age group we assessed. The language used in the items also did not seem to be too difficult (e.g., "My mother respects my feelings"; "I wish I had a different mother"; "I can count on my mother to listen to my problems"). However, the original had five response categories from *never* to *always*, which we reduced to three choices in order to make it easier for younger children to answer.

We also included two measures of parentification. First, we created parallel 21-item scales for the mother's and child's perceptions of the child's adult role taking and responsibilities. We adapted items from the Parentification Scale (Mika, Bergner, & Baum, 1987), which is a 30-item tool originally developed for college students. The scale asked about household responsibilities (e.g., cleaning, doing the dishes) and about being an adviser, consoler, or confidant to one's parent or siblings. Respondents rated each item on a 5-point scale from *never* to *very often*. We omitted items on the child's role in interactions between parents because our study included mostly single-mother households, which resulted in two 21-item scales. Second, we used a modified version of the Emotional Parentification Questionnaire (Martin, 1996). This 18-item tool measures the degree to which the child serves as a caregiver to and is emotionally supportive of the mother and it also was originally created for college students. We reduced the original 5-point Likert response scale to 4 points, simplified the wording on some questions, and created a parallel version for mothers.

Data Analyses

In comparing responses from study participants in HIV-affected and unaffected households, the significance tests used for categorical data were chi-square tests; t tests were used to compare mean scores. Pearson correlations were used to examine the strength of relationships between continuous variables. Multiple regression also was used to investigate the relationships of independent variables to the dependent variable, controlling for other possible confounders.

RESULTS

Study Sample

The characteristics of the total sample reflect the demography of New York City. Approximately 57% of mothers were Black and 39% were Latina; the average age of the index child was 12; and 28% of the children were male. Of the mothers, 73% were single and almost 40% had less than a high school education. The sample of mothers with HIV/AIDS and their children was generally similar to mothers and children in the "well" comparison group in background characteristics (see Table 1.1).

Our first important observation from the study data was that many of the inner-city mothers had health problems other than HIV/AIDS that could lead to child caregiving. Almost one third of the comparison sample of mothers reported having an ongoing chronic health condition that caused them to spend days in bed, be hospitalized, or have an activity restriction. Their conditions included epilepsy, diabetes, asthma, hypothyroidism,

Table 1.1		
Sample Characteristics		
Characteristic	HIV	Well
Mean age of mother (years)	38	37
Mean age of index child (years)	13	12
Black (%)	61	51
Hispanic (%)	33	46
Single mothers (%)	72	73
High school graduates (%)	59	65
Male index child (%)	36	16

and rheumatic fever. There were too few of these mothers to permit formal statistical analyses, but inspection of the data showed that these mothers had rates of disability related to health problems similar to those of the mothers with HIV/AIDS. Furthermore, children in these families were called on to perform caregiving tasks of a similar scope, responsibility, and consequence as children in HIV/AIDS families. We decided to exclude the mothers with serious health conditions from the comparison sample and conducted the balance of the analysis on the 51 mothers with HIV/AIDS and 36 well mothers in the community sample, that is, mothers who did not report a serious chronic health condition.

Type and Frequency of Child Caregiving

The first aim of our study was to document the extent to which children take on adult responsibilities when a parent has HIV/AIDS. This section outlines the types and extent of care that mothers and children reported.

Personal Care

We found that a majority of children said they had performed personal care tasks when their mother was ill, but few performed them regularly. More than 8 in 10 children overall said they had "ever" helped by feeding, bathing, or dressing their mother or by assisting her in getting around the house and 21% reported having helped with all four personal tasks. More than one in five reported that they helped their mother "a lot" with one or more personal care tasks. There were no differences between children with well or HIV-affected mothers in the child reports (see Table 1.2). Similarly, on the Parentification Scale item that asked about child provision of personal care—"child is responsible for the care of the mother when she is sick"—neither child nor mother reports differed between the HIV and well comparison groups (see Table 1.3).

We also determined that children of mothers with HIV/AIDS spend many more hours providing personal care to their mothers than children of healthy parents, both in a typical week and especially when the mother is ill. In a typical week, mothers with HIV reported that their child spent

Table 1.2

Child Reports of Providing Personal Care to the Mother

Personal care task	Children who provided this kind of care "ever" or "a lot" (%)		Children who provided this kind of care "a lot" (%)	
	Mother with HIV	Well mother	Mother with HIV	Well mother
Feeding	66	66	10	9
Getting around the house	69	71	19	12
Getting dressed	49	57	7	6
Bathing	33	34	2	0

6.2 hours providing personal care compared with 1.2 hours reported in the well sample ($p = .05$). Four children were reported to spend more than 16 hours caring for their mother in a typical week. These figures were much higher when mothers with HIV were sick compared with when unaffected mothers were sick: 13.3 versus 3.0 hours per week ($p < .005$). When mothers were sick, more children provided personal care: 66% of

Table 1.3

Mother and Child Reports: Percentages of Children and Mothers Who Said the Child Is Responsible for the Care of the Mother When She Is Sick

Response	Children reporting (%)		Mothers reporting (%)	
	HIV	Well	HIV	Well
Never	20	23	43	46
Rarely	10	9	20	24
Occasionally	30	20	18	5
Often	26	29	8	16
Very often	12	20	12	5

children spent time caring for their mother, and 11 children were reported to spend more than 16 hours per week caring for their sick mother.

Sibling Care

Of the 87 children in the two groups, 33 had no siblings, so reports for this kind of caregiving are based on 54 children, 32 in the HIV-affected group and 22 in the well-mother group. Overall, 64% of children reported having "ever" cared for their siblings, with 19% saying they provided care "a lot." Caring for siblings is a common task that children have in families, whether a parent has HIV or not. However, when parents have HIV/AIDS, children spend more time caring for siblings on a routine basis, and especially when the mother is ill. Mothers with HIV/AIDS reported that in a typical week, children provided 8.7 hours of care on average for siblings, more than those in well families (4.7 hours). However, when the mother was ill, the amount of time children of HIV-affected mothers spent providing care to siblings increased to 18.7 hours on average versus 7.1 by children in unaffected households.

Household Responsibilities

We asked about four household tasks that children often do in a home: laundry, grocery shopping, cooking, and household cleaning. Child and mother reports of the types of chores done by children did not differ between the HIV and well groups (see Table 1.4). In both groups, when the mother was ill, children spent more time on household chores: Mothers reported that in a typical week, children spent an average of 3.5 hours performing household chores compared with 4.6 hours per week spent when the mother was sick. There also was a marked discrepancy between mothers' and children's reports of these chores: Mothers were more likely than children to report that their children never did chores around the house. For example, 82% of children reported that they had some responsibility for at least one household task compared with only 73% of mothers. Mothers and children agreed, however, that children rarely had "usual" responsibility for any chore. The Parentification Scale also had

Table 1.4

Disparity Between Mother and Child Reports About Performance of Household Tasks

Report	Child report (%)		Mother report (%)	
	HIV	Well	HIV	Well
Child never makes dinner	26	39	51	60
Child never cleans up for family	8	19	35	35
Child never washes dishes	8	14	22	30

three items that addressed household responsibility—whether the child makes dinner, cleans up, or does dishes for the family. The mean score on a subscale formed from these items was 8.9 for children and 6.5 for their mothers, showing again that parents were less likely to report that children performed these tasks than the children.

Emotional Support

When mothers were asked to name people who provided emotional support (e.g., people whom they confided in, who really understood their life), 22% of mothers with HIV/AIDS named the index child compared with 14% of mothers who were well. This was not a statistically significant difference. We found little difference between groups on the two measures of emotional parentification that the mothers and children completed. On the Emotional Parentification subscale of the Parentification Scale, neither mother reports (13.0 vs. 12.0) nor child reports (15.1 vs. 14.3) were significantly different. The same was true for maternal reports on the Emotional Parentification Questionnaire (18.4 vs. 17.1) and child reports (19.6 vs. 19.9).

Which Children Assume Caregiving Responsibilities?

The second study aim was to identify which children were more likely to become child caregivers. We examined whether age and gender were related to measures of each kind of care using multiple regression and found, contrary to our hypothesis, that in general, girls and older children were not more likely than other children to report taking on personal care tasks, household tasks, or sibling care. However, mothers reported that older children did have more household tasks to perform than younger children both in general and when the mother was ill. On the provision of emotional support, results were more in line with our hypothesis that girls were more likely to be named as a supporter to their mothers than boys ($\beta = .22$, $p = .05$), but age was unrelated.

Younger children also reported doing more personal care tasks for their mothers than older children did. This is part of a larger pattern in which younger children's own self-reports consistently presented themselves as providing more care and emotional support. This pattern of findings suggests that younger children may be interpreting certain questions on the questionnaire as a "test" of their affection and helpfulness to their mothers, and that they may be underreporting their problems, overreporting their responsibilities, or both under- and overreporting their problems or responsibilities. The sample size was too small to permit further statistical analysis of this cluster. We also examined whether child caregiving was less frequent or intense when there was an older sibling in the household or an adult present. However, having an older person in the house was not a protective factor—children provided the same amount of care either way.

Correlates of Being a Caregiver for Children

Our third aim was to describe the correlates of filling the caregiving role for children. Our findings follow.

Perceptions About Child's Level of Responsibility

As noted above, we measured the perceptions of both mothers and children about whether the child had too much responsibility around the house or had to give things up (see Table 1.5). Mothers in the HIV group were less likely to feel that the child could handle all of his or her chores

Table 1.5

Maternal and Child Reports: Perceptions About Child's Responsibility for Household Chores

	Child reporting "very true" or "somewhat true" (%)		Mother reporting "very true" or "somewhat true" (%)	
Report	HIV	Well	HIV	Well
Child has too much responsibility	45	44	6	16
Child has to give things up	49	36	16	14
Child can handle chores	90	92	78	95
Mother appreciates what child does	96	91	96	100
Mother complains about what child does	44	67	61	46
Child is more capable because of chores	88	94	82	92

($p < .05$), but the groups did not differ significantly on any other maternal ratings. Among children, the only significant difference was that children of well mothers were more likely to report that the mother complained about what they did around the house ($p < .05$). In both groups, children who said they provided "a lot" of personal care to their mothers did not see themselves as more burdened than other children. When parents and children differed from each other, the children reported more negative consequences from having household duties than their mothers did, including having too much responsibility and giving things up to do chores.

Perceptions About Whether Tasks Interfered With Child's Activities

Children also were asked whether their household responsibilities interfered with other things they needed or wanted to do (homework, participation in after school activities, watching TV, or spending time with friends). Overall, 87% reported that their chores did interfere with at least one activity. However, only 14% said their chores "always" interfered with an activity. Most children reported that chores interfered with time spent with friends or watching TV; few reported that chores interfered with homework or after school activities. The same pattern occurred when children were asked how things were different when the parent was ill. Although more reported some interference with activities, most of the interference was in peer relationships and TV watching.

Perceptions of Mental Health

Another part of our third aim was to describe the mental health of children in the caregiving role, particularly rates of depression, conduct problems, or other types of emotional disturbance. These are described in the following sections.

Children's self-rated depression. Children of mothers with HIV/ AIDS rated their depression on the CDI about the same as children in the well sample (6.8 vs. 7.1, *ns*). About 20% of children scored above the cutoff of 11 on the CDI, which indicates clinically significant symptoms. This is twice the rate found in community-based studies of children. No significant relationships were found between type or degree of caregiving and child-reported depression on the CDI. Children who had more personal care, household task, and sibling care responsibilities did not have higher self-reported depression scores. We also found no relationship between reporting that chores interfered with usual activities and CDI scores.

Counter to our hypothesis, children who were named as providing emotional support to their mothers did not have higher depression scores than those not named (6.8 vs. 7.0, *ns*). In fact, the opposite was true: Children whose scores were higher on the Emotional Parentification Questionnaire had lower depression scores ($-.21, p < .05$); the same pattern was true for the Emotional Parentification subscale of the Parentification scale ($-.20, p = .05$). We had also hypothesized that having an older sibling or an adult present in the home would be a protective factor—that is, that child caregivers with older siblings would be less likely to be depressed. However, this was not the case: Having an older sibling or adult in the household was not associated with lower depression scores.

Children's self-rated behavior. Children aged 11 and older ($n = 55$) completed the YSR. The average score on the YSR was 49.5, which approximates the mean found in normative samples (Achenbach, 1991b). Fifteen percent of children scored above the clinical cutoff, which indicates clinically significant behavioral problems. Children of parents with HIV had the same mean score on the YSR as children of well mothers. Because of this, we combined them for the next analysis.

Children's self-reported behavioral problems were unrelated to providing sibling care or emotional support to the mother. However, children who typically provided more personal care to mothers (on a routine basis rather just when the mother was sick) had more behavior problems (internalizing and externalizing). Also, the more time children spent on household tasks when a parent was ill, the higher the reports of internalizing symptoms ($r = .21, p = .10$).

Parental reports of behavioral problems. The mean CBCL score in this sample was 50.7, similar to the scale's normative samples (Achenbach, 1991a), but 20% of children in this sample scored above the cutoff of 63 (indicative of clinical symptoms), twice community norms. Children of mothers with HIV/AIDS tended to have higher scores than children of well mothers on the internalizing (51.7 vs. 47.4, $p = .07$) and externalizing subscales (51.7 vs. 48.4, $p = .16$) as well as on the total score (52.0 vs. 47.7, $p = .11$), but none of the differences reached formal statistical significance.

Overall, children's caregiving responsibilities (in any domain) were never related to higher CBCL scores. However, children who were named by mothers as providing emotional support tended to have lower internalizing and externalizing scores on the CBCL, which suggests that parents choose to confide in children who have fewer behavioral symptoms.

Parent–child relationship. There were no differences between the two groups on parent–child relationships as reported by either mothers using the CBQ or children on the IPPA. Thus, this resource for children, that is, the parent–child relationship, was not compromised by the parents' HIV/AIDS. However, being a provider of emotional support to the mother was correlated with child ratings of the relationship; overall, the better (lower) the child's score on the parent–child relationship scale, the higher their scores on the Emotional Parentification Questionnaire ($r = -.29$, $p < .01$) and the Emotional Parentification subscale ($r = -.19$, $p < .05$). Thus, similar to findings for parent-rated adjustment scores on the CBCL, mothers may choose the children with whom they feel they have the best relationships as the ones they share things with and talk to like adults about their problems.

DISCUSSION

Child caregiving is a developmental anomaly. Little has been documented about how often or to what extent school-aged children act as caregivers to their parents, and we tend to assume that children placed in this unnatural role will experience serious effects on their development and well-being. In our study, we attempted to answer several important questions about the children who participated: How often are children their parents' caregivers? Which children are likely to be caregivers? What constitutes the well-being of children who have this responsibility? We also examined whether the answers were influenced by the mother's HIV/AIDS status. What we found was that caregiving is a frequent responsibility of school-aged children; that they are called on to perform a variety of caregiving tasks from extra chores to toileting; and that some spend many hours a week in the caregiving role, especially when the parent is ill. Although parents and children sometimes disagree about the extent of the child's responsibilities and chores, there is little question that parents rely on their children for help and that children provide that help.

We also found that despite a high caregiving load, few children perceived serious consequences from their work, and there was little evidence of serious mental health correlates. This is surprising, given the large number of children affected and the high demand of caregiving in HIV-affected families. For example, a majority of children, even those in families unaffected by HIV/AIDS, have performed personal care tasks when their mothers were ill. Children of mothers with HIV/AIDS spend many more hours providing personal care to their mothers than children of healthy parents, both in a typical week and especially when the mother is ill.

Children also become part of their parent's support network. Children whose mothers have HIV/AIDS provide support at about the same rate as children of healthy mothers. Although we feared that children burdened with their parents' fears of disability, death, poverty, and abandonment might suffer depression or anxiety, we found no evidence of this in this sample.

We also failed to support commonly held hypotheses about which children in a household might experience the caregiver role. Within this sample of 8- to 16-year-olds, no consistent evidence demonstrated that older children or girls were more likely to take on personal care, household maintenance, or sibling caregiving responsibilities, although mothers did report that older children did a greater number of tasks both usually and when they were sick. Girls were more likely to provide emotional support to their mothers than boys were.

So how were children affected by caregiving responsibilities? Over one half reported having too much responsibility, and children in general reported that their household responsibilities interfered with their spending time with friends and watching TV. However, mothers in general did not think children had too many chores, which we believe is a healthy echo of conversations about chores between children and their parents in most American households. Parents did admit that when they were sick, their children spent more time on chores, but the overwhelming majority were confident that their children could handle all their household chores and were more capable because of them.

Mental health problems are not an inevitable consequence of child caregiving, although some situations warrant attention. Children of mothers with HIV/AIDS rated their own depressive symptoms and behavior problems and their relationships with their mothers about the same as children of unaffected mothers. Child caregivers—those who had more personal care, household task, and sibling care responsibilities— did not have higher self-reported depression scores. Self-reported behavioral problems also were unrelated to providing sibling care or emotional support to the mother. However, behavior problems were both more frequent or more severe or both in children who provided personal care on a regular basis and in those who took on household chores when the mother was ill.

The developmental concern for child caregivers is parentification. An extensive literature documents poor mental health among children who care for parents with mental health and drug or alcohol problems, but little research has explored the effects of parental physical health problems and parentification. Contrary to our expectation, depression symptoms were lower among children who experienced higher emotional parentification, and children who provided emotional support tended to have fewer behavioral problems. Similarly, we found higher emotional parentification scores in families where the mother or child rated their relationship as closer and more secure. Because this was a cross-sectional survey, we cannot determine the direction of this relationship, but we believe that taken together, these findings suggest that mothers may choose a well-adjusted child to become a caregiver.

Children in our sample had higher than average depression scores. This may be related more to the fact that children lived in poor, inner-city families than to the fact of their extra responsibilities as child caregivers. Thus, much as expressed within life span development theory, context plays an important part in development. Our research shows that the context of this study is important. Both the types of responsibilities assigned to children and the positive and negative impact of caregiving on their development may be different in other populations.

It is important to note the study's limitations. Because the sample size is fairly small, we were unable to analyze differences between subgroups of children having sick or well parents, such as boys versus girls. There also were too few parents in the comparison sample who had other types of chronic health conditions to analyze them as a separate category. It is difficult to trust statistical significance tests under these circumstances; therefore, we see this study as an exploratory effort. It is important that this research be replicated with a larger sample to better test for these trends and to permit more detailed research on subgroups such as younger children and girls. In addition, the study sample is not a random sample and may not be representative.

In contrast, a study strength was that in reporting about child mental health, the parent–child relationship, and how often children take on caregiving responsibilities in each category, we included both mother and child reports rather than relying on a single rater. As a result, one critical observation we made was that in general, children reported that they did many more tasks around the house than their mothers reported. In the child mental health literature, agreement between parents and children has been well studied, and it has been suggested that differences in their responses are more likely to be due to the uniquely different information held by the reporters than to a lack of validity in the responses of either rater (Karver, 2006). Agreement across sources also tends to be low to moderate when assessing other domains, such as family functioning or physical health (Holmbeck, Li, Schurman, Friedman, & Coakley, 2002). It is important to recognize that there is a universal discrepancy in perceptions between mothers and children and to obtain information from both when assessing degree of caregiving provided by children. We would like to better understand the nature and reasons for the discrepant reports between parents and children. We therefore recommend that further research be conducted to identify reporting bias, examine social desirability, and evaluate the validity of parentification measures with younger children.

This study provides room for optimism about the effects on children of caregiving responsibilities, but given the study's limitations, we recommend further in-depth study of the needs of child caregivers. We also recommend that preventive and supportive intervention programs be considered for children in the caregiving role. Although our study does not document consistent negative effects, children themselves certainly perceive negative effects, particularly on leisure activities. More important, some with routine caregiver responsibilities reported elevated psychological symptoms. Preventive interventions are universal by design and seek to strengthen children through providing developmentally appropriate skills and adult mentors to support them. The goal is to help maintain and increase resilience in these children, who are experiencing a stressful life event that is developmentally unusual, the serious illness and possible death of a parent. We believe that community-based programs for families in which a parent is ill can perform several important functions. First, they can be a safety net and rescue child caregivers facing emergencies such as financial and food insufficiency, medical emergencies, or cognitive impairments in parents who do not recognize their limitations. Second, they can help parents and children communicate their expectations of the child caregiver more clearly and can help family members reconcile their disparate opinions about the extent to which children take on responsibilities in the household. Third, they can connect families to existing services that parents are too ill to identify and children are too unskilled to find. Fourth, they can monitor the mental health of children in these high-risk families and identify children who experience elevated symptoms.

Our research would be more easily interpretable if we knew more about the roles of children in average households. Although there have been a few studies in the past 2 decades that have examined the amount of time that U.S. children spend on housework, scholars still do not agree on whether theses duties are harmful or helpful to children's social and cognitive development (Lee et al., 2003). Moreover, children whose parents are seriously ill with conditions such as AIDS may have a range of responsibilities in addition to the usual household tasks. They may assume household duties typically performed by adults and sometimes be called on to provide personal care or emotional support to the ill parent. Because little is known about the emotional consequences that children face in living with the stresses of these added responsibilities, continued research to learn about the typical outcomes among child caregivers is essential.

By 2010, more than 40 million children in 34 countries hardest hit by HIV/AIDS will have suffered the illness and death of a parent (Hunter & Williamson, 2000). Around the world, many children live with an HIV-infected adult in need of medical care. Many of these children become caregivers to ill parents with HIV/AIDS for some time before parental death, and they may face premature termination of schooling, take on personal care and household responsibilities normally considered appropriate for adults, or undertake outside paid labor. Younger children may be raised by older siblings or left without regular supervision. Our work in New York needs to be replicated in the world's developing countries, which bear an unequal burden of HIV/AIDS.

REFERENCES

Achenbach, T. (1991a). *Manual for the Child Behavior Checklist/4–18 and 1991 profile*. Burlington: Department of Psychiatry, University of Vermont.

Achenbach, T. (1991b). *Manual for the Youth Self-Report and 1991 profile*. Burlington: Department of Psychiatry, University of Vermont.

Armsden, C., & Greenberg, M. T. (1987). The inventory of parent and peer attachment: Individual differences and their relationship to psychological well-being in adolescence. *Journal of Youth and Adolescence, 16,* 427–454.

Baltes, P. B., Lindenberger, U., & Staudinger, U. M. (1998). Life-span theory in developmental psychology. In R. M. Lerner (Ed.), *Handbook of child psychology: Vol. 1. Theoretical models of human development* (pp. 1029–1143). New York: Wiley.

Barnett, B., & Parker, G. (1998). The parentified child: Early competence or childhood deprivation? *Child Psychology and Psychiatry Review, 3,* 146–166.

Barreto, S., & McManus, M. (1997). Casting the net for "depression" among ethnic minority children from the high-risk urban communities. *Clinical Psychology Review, 17,* 823–845.

Bauman, L. J., Foster, G., Silver, E. J., Gamble, I., & Muchaneta, L. (2006). Children care for their ill parents with HIV/AIDS. *Vulnerable Children and Youth Studies, 1,* 56–70.

Bauman, L. J., Phuong, L., Silver, E. J., & Berman, R. (2001, May). *Lean on me? Adjustment of children who provide support to their ill mothers with HIV/AIDS.* Paper presented at the 41st Meeting of the Ambulatory Pediatrics Association, Baltimore.

Becker, S. (October 2003–April 2004). Carers. *Research Matters, 16,* 11–16.

Becker, S., & Dearden, C. (October 2004–April 2005). Carers. *Research Matters, 18,* 11–18.

Cates, J., Graham, L., Boeglin, D., & Tiekler, S. (1990). The effect of AIDS on the family system. *Families in Society: The Journal of Contemporary Human Services, 7,* 195–201.

Eccles, J. S. (1999). The development of children ages 6 to 14. *The Future of Children, 9,* 30–44.

Elkind, D. (2001). *The hurried child: Growing up too fast too soon.* Cambridge, MA: De Capo Press.

Holmbeck, G. N., Li, S. T., Schurman, J. V., Friedman, D., & Coakley, R. M. (2002). Collecting and managing multisource and multimethod data in studies of pediatric populations. *Journal of Pediatric Psychology, 27,* 5–18.

Hunt, G., Levine, C., & Naiditch, L. (2005). *Young caregivers in the U.S.: Findings from a national survey.* Bethesda, MD: National Alliance on Caregiving.

Hunter, S., & Williamson, J. (2000). *Children on the brink 2000*. Washington, DC: U.S. Agency for International Development.

Ilfeld, F. (1976). Further validation of a psychiatric symptom index in a normal population. *Psychological Reports, 39,* 1215–1228.

Karver, M. S. (2006). Determinants of multiple informant agreement on child and adolescent behavior. *Journal of Abnormal Child Psychology, 34,* 251–262.

Kovacs, M. (1985). The Children's Depression Inventory (CDI). *Psychopharmacology Bulletin, 21,* 995–998.

Kovacs, M. (1992). *The Children's Depression Inventory, manual.* Toronto, Ontario, Canada: Multi-Health Systems.

Lee, Y., Schneider, B., & Waite, L. J. (2003). Children and housework: Some unanswered questions. *Sociological Studies of Children and Youth, 9,* 105–125.

Levine, C. (1990). AIDS and changing concepts of family. *Milbank Quarterly, 68,* 33–59.

Levine, C. (1995). Orphans of the HIV epidemic. Unmet needs in six U.S. cities. *AIDS Care, 7*(Suppl. 1), S57–S62.

Levine, M. D. (1999). Middle childhood. In M. D. Levine, W. B. Carey, & A. C. Crocker (Eds.). *Developmental–behavioral pediatrics* (pp. 51–67). Philadelphia: Saunders.

Martin, M. T. (1996). Mother–daughter relations in divorced families: Parentification and internalizing and relationship problems. *Dissertation Abstracts International: Section B: The Sciences & Engineering, 56*(9-B), 5176.

Mika, P., Bergner, R. M., & Baum, M. C. (1987). The development of a scale for the assessment of parentification. *Family Therapy, 3,* 229–235.

Papalia, D. E., Olds, S. W., & Feldman, R. D. (2007). *Human development* (10th ed.). New York: McGraw-Hill.

Prinz, R. J., Foster, R., Kent, R. N., & O'Leary, K. D. (1979). Multivariate assessment of conflict in distressed and nondistressed mother–adolescent dyads. *Journal of Applied Behavior Analysis, 12,* 691–700.

Robin, A., & Foster, S. (1989). Questionnaire and observation assessment. In A. Robin & S. Foster (Eds.), *Negotiating parent–adolescent conflict* (pp. 77–98). New York: Guilford Press.

Robson, E. (2000). Invisible carers: Young people in Zimbabwe's home-based healthcare. *Area, 32,* 59–69.

Robson, E. (2004). Hidden child workers: Young carers in Zimbabwe. *Antipode, 36,* 227–248.

Siskowski, C. (2004). *Middle school responses to family health outcomes: The effects of family caregiving on the education of middle school students with family health issues.* Unpublished doctoral dissertation, Lynn University, Boca Raton, FL.

Smucker, M. R., Craighead, W. E., Craighead, L. W., & Green, B. (1986). Normative and reliability data for the Children's Depression Inventory. *Journal of Abnormal Child Psychology, 14,* 25–39.

Stein, J., Riedel, M., & Rotheram-Borus, M. (1999). Parentification and its impact on adolescent children of parents with AIDS. *Family Process, 38,* 193–208.

Thomas, N., Stainton, T., Jackson, S., Cheung, W., Doubtfire, S., & Webb, A. (2003). "Your friends don't understand": Invisibility and unmet need in the lives of "young carers." *Child and Family Social Work, 8,* 35–46.

Tompkins, T. L. (2007). Parentification and maternal HIV infection: Beneficial role or pathological burden? *Journal of Child and Family Studies, 16,* 113–125.

Wallace, B. (1996). *Adult children of dysfunctional families: Prevention, intervention, and treatment for community mental health promotion.* Westport, CT: Praeger.

2

Adolescent Caregivers

Connie Siskowski

One of the key principles of life span development—that development is dependent on history and context—is important for understanding the increasing numbers and growing importance of adolescent caregivers in U.S. society. Recent U.S. history includes significant developments in medicine and technology that allow people to live longer. People are now more likely to survive accidents and illnesses and live at home rather than in a care facility (National Center for Health Statistics, 2007). Longevity, illness, and disability, although obviously affecting one's ability to engage in the activities of daily living, also change the dynamics of the caregiving situation. Older people and persons living with illness and disability are frequently unable to lead fully independent lives and thus require assistance with daily activities.

Changes in family structure over time include more single-parent households and more grandparents, whose health may be failing, either living in an intergenerational household or having guardianship responsibilities for grandchildren. More people in the same household are employed, thus having less time available for caregiving. These changes have resulted in adolescents becoming the silent, hidden, and unrecognized providers of care when family health situations arise.

When a family health issue creates dependence on another for care or support, adolescents placed in a caregiver role move beyond what is normally expected of them. Adolescents take on adult roles within the family and assume responsibilities for which they have little or no preparation.

The teen's burdens and stresses are typically overlooked by health and education professionals as well as by family and community.

The purpose of this chapter is to discuss the effects of the caregiver role on adolescents during these formative years. I begin by summarizing the available statistics on adolescent caregivers in the United States. Second, I discuss development in adolescence and how developmental experiences may be affected by taking on the caregiving role. Third, I present U.S. and international research on adolescent caregivers. Finally, I present findings from the first study on the effects of caregiving in adolescence in Palm Beach County, Florida, the What Works Survey (B. Miller, Bunker, & Kelley-Miller, 2003).

STATISTICS ON ADOLESCENT CAREGIVERS

Research revealing the prevalence of young caregivers in the United States and the effects that caregiving has on them is growing (Beach, 1997; Gates & Lackey, 1998; Orel & Dupuy, 2002; Shifren, 2001; Siskowski, 2003, 2004, 2006a, 2006c; National Alliance for Caregiving & The United Hospital Fund [NAC & UHF], 2005). As stated in chapter 1, this volume, the first U.S. national survey on caregiving youth contained population estimates that at least 1.3 million to 1.4 million children and adolescents between the ages of 8 and 18 years fulfill family caregiving responsibilities (NAC & UHF, 2005). Of the survey's sample of 213 caregiving youth, nearly half (49%) reported spending "a lot of time" caregiving; many young caregivers tended to live in single-parent and lower income households, and 38% cared for a grandparent (NAC & UHF, 2005).

Individuals under 18 years of age now account for about 26% of the U.S. population, far less than the 1964 baby boomer peak of 36% (Federal Interagency Forum on Child and Family Statistics, 2000). Four million U.S. young people have developmental disabilities and another 10 million have chronic illnesses, of whom nearly 10% require significant medical support services (Lamorey, 1999). These youth are likely to have siblings who share in helping with their care and support.

It is likely that the estimate of caregiving children in the United States is conservative. The 2004 report *Caregiving in the U.S.* (National Alliance for Caregiving & American Association of Retired Persons [NAC & AARP], 2004) estimated that there are 22.9 million caregiving households in which 37% of participants (8.5 million) also have youth under the age of 18 years living at home. The report does not and was never intended to provide information about the ages of these youth; roles they assume; or effects of family caregiving on their lives, including developmental issues, socialization, and education. Furthermore, this report excluded families in which the primary caregiver was a youth.

The effects of poverty and race are important aspects of the statistics on adolescent caregivers. They influence both positive and negative aspects of development for adolescent caregivers, just as they do for noncaregivers.

Race and Adolescent Caregivers

The extent of ethnic and racial diversity is greater than ever in America. The most dramatic population increase has been among Hispanics: The Hispanic youth population increased from 9% in 1980 to 16% in 2000 (Federal Interagency Forum on Child and Family Statistics, 2000). Among caregivers with youth under age 18 years in their households who participated in the NAC and AARP (2004, p. 27) national survey, 53% were Black, in contrast with 39% Hispanic, 35% Caucasian, and 34% Asian, and future population increases among minority older adults have been projected (Williams, 2002). Although the Caucasian elderly population has a lower prevalence of functional deficits, it has a higher rate of facility care than the minority elderly population (Sahyoun, Pratt, Lentzner, Dey, & Robinson, 2001; U.S. Department of Health & Human Services, 1998). This implies that minority populations utilize more home-based care than the general population overall; however, little is known about the intensity or the tribulations of this care (Dilworth-Anderson, Williams, & Cooper, 1999).

Young Caregivers in the U.S. (NAC & UHF, 2005) reported that according to their parents, caregivers from minority households who were 12 to 18 years of age scored higher on measures of anxiety and depression as well as antisocial behavior than their counterparts from nonminority households. Young caregivers also reported more recent sadness within the past week (69% minority vs. 47% nonminority) and felt that there was no use in letting their feelings show (33% vs. 15%). The report shows that the minority households were less likely to have outside help with caregiving tasks, which may help explain why minority youth more frequently reported experiencing the negative ramifications of caregiving.

The challenge is accentuated for minorities when increased requirements for home care are combined with more health care disparities from the general population, which are potentially further complicated by language barriers. Difficulties in communication may occur in the delivery of health care and with family members who assist with caregiving. The U.S. census of 2000 documented that there were 10 million persons who did not speak English and 20 million who spoke English poorly (U.S. Census Bureau, 2001). The role of adolescent caregivers in such families may include verbal and written translation.

Poverty and Adolescent Caregivers

Poverty not only increases the liklihood of the need for care, it also decreases the ability to pay privately for help with home care. Furthermore, persons who are at lower income levels with average wages of less than $15 per hour have fewer benefits and less time off than workers earning average wages greater than $15 per hour (U.S. Department of Labor, 2006). Poor health, whether short or long term, also increases demands for family caregiving. In the absence of public programs, an inability to pay for in-home assistance decreases available options for support, relief, and help for both the one in need of care and the family caregiver.

Public support systems for family caregivers, especially for adult caregivers under age 60 years, unless they are caring for an adult over the age of 60 years, and child caregivers are typically unavailable. The National Family Caregiver Support Program, a federal program first authorized in December 2000 and renewed each year, is attached to the Older Americans Act and administered by the U.S. Administration on Aging (U.S. Department of Health & Human Services, 2004). New legislation, the Lifespan Respite Care Act, which, if funding appropriations are made, will be of help to caregivers of all ages, effective in 2009.

Poverty is more common among persons who are older and who are members of a minority. Nearly 14% of people who are at least 85 years of age live below the poverty threshold. Of the older Black population, 22% are poor, and nearly 19% of Hispanics fall in this poverty class (Butler, 2001). Research validates that ethnic minorities who provide care at home have a lower income, are more often single, and are more frequently younger than peers who are Caucasian (Knight, Silverstein, McCallum, & Fox, 2000). Any one of these factors—age, poverty, minority status—compounds the likelihood of both health risks and young caregivers.

Despite the evidence that increasing numbers of adolescents are taking on the caregiving role for family members, most U.S. research has focused only on the effects of caring for a family member on the adult family caregiver. The typical family caregiver is portrayed as a married employed woman who assists her mother who does not live with her (NAC & AARP, 2004). Studies have shown the physical, psychological, and financial effects on the family caregiver related to this extended, and in some cases uninvited, role (Kiecolt-Glaser et al. 2003; Schulz & Beach, 1999; Wang, 2005).

DEVELOPMENTAL EXPERIENCES FOR ADOLESCENT CAREGIVERS AND NONCAREGIVERS

To understand the effects of the adolescent caregiving role on development, and vice versa, one must understand normal development during adolescence. I next discuss normal developmental tasks of adolescence and how these tasks affect and are affected by the caregiving role. When possible, comparisons between adolescent caregivers and noncaregivers are provided.

In addition to the challenges of caring for persons who are unable to care for themselves, adolescents are dealing with normal developmental growth and change. Biological development during adolescence includes the onset of puberty, and puberty brings substantial hormonal, physical, and cognitive changes that may make coping with the health condition of a relative difficult (Worsham & Crawford, 2005).

Chapter 1 of this volume discusses some changes in cognitive development during adolescence, including the development of formal operational thought. For cognitive development to progress at a normal rate, adolescents need exposure to materials that stimulate thinking and contemplation of ideas. Obviously, the academic environment provides most opportunities in this realm, and when 1 in 5 young caregivers report that caregiving has made them miss school or after-school activities and 15% say that it has made them miss homework (NAC & UHF, 2005), it is likely that some opportunities are missed. Adolescent caregivers may be able to compensate for lost academic opportunities by enriched learning experiences with the care recipient at home. In much the same way as the workplace allows telecommuting to retain adult family caregivers, perhaps distance learning could be an option for students who must give care at home.

Many changes in psychosocial development occur during the adolescent period. Adolescents must deal with the angst of adolescence—peer pressure; attitudes toward parents; and acceptance of their own appearance, abilities or disabilities, society, and environment (N. B. Miller & Sammons, 1999). Furthermore, it is a time when youth are "most likely to experiment with at-risk behaviors" (National Middle School Association, 2003, p. 1) such as smoking and drinking.

Individuals from 12 to 14 years old (early adolescence) need to learn emotional independence from family, and they seek acceptance by peers. In studies of early adolescents dealing with parental cancer, time designed to be with peers and further their independent thinking and behavioral processes was reported to conflict with caregiving responsibilities and the need to be physically and emotionally at home (Davey & Davey, 2005; Faulkner & Davey, 2002). During later adolescence (ages 15 to 17), teens emotionally separate further from family and are better able to understand the implications of illness (Rizzo & Kirkland, 2005). For example, they realize that instead of going away to college they may need to consider the choice of remaining at home or going to college close by to continue to be of assistance to their family.

The development of identity and ego is important in a youth's passage through adolescence (Erikson, 1968). Adolescents question and explore their own beliefs, values, personal characteristics, and sexuality. Identity development is lifelong, but much change in identity development is considered normal during the adolescent period because adolescents experience rapid changes in biology and social relationships. Beach's (1997) study on adolescent caregivers discussed research by adolescent specialists and postulated that when families come together to deal with a caregiving situation, such as a person with Alzheimer's disease living within the family unit, there may be a delay in the identity development of the adolescent (Beach, 1997).

Feelings about self-worth among caregivers have been studied in comparison with noncaregiving samples. The NAC and UHF (2005) survey reveals that caregiving children 12 to 18 years old feel worthless or inferior and are more prone to sudden changes in mood compared with noncaregiving children in the same age group. Caregivers also exhibit more antisocial behavior than noncaregivers, are more likely to have trouble getting along with teachers, are more likely to be bullies, and are more likely to associate with kids who tend to get into trouble.

Perhaps some of these differences can be attributed to the stressors these adolescents face as young caregivers, stressors that just increase "normal" stressors of adolescent development, one example being school transitions. School transitions can affect social development or academic performance in adolescents (Eccles, 2004). Students in the 1st year of middle school are in transition, having left the cocoon of elementary school. At this time, and then again in high school, these young caregivers meet children from many schools, perhaps even from several towns. The effect of school transition has not been studied in adolescent caregivers, so specific comparisons with noncaregivers cannot be made.

With increased academic, social, and personal demands on their lives, adolescents must learn to accept new forms of responsibility. Housework is one such responsibility that most adolescents take on. Adolescent caregivers perform increasing amounts of household chores (Lackey & Gates, 2001). In relation to household tasks, one report suggested that when children understand the necessity of their role, they view it as positive (Goodnow, 1988). Miriam from Nebraska (American Association of Caregiving Youth, n.d.), who was a National Multiple Sclerosis Society scholarship winner, wrote, "My mom's MS has made me a more responsible person. I am at the top of my class and I plan to pursue a career in medicine." A Florida high school senior who was caring for his disabled father while his mother worked stated in a scholarship application,

> Some might look at Dad's limitations and think about how much they have to give up to provide for his care but I believe that this is an amazing opportunity for me to strengthen our relationship and teach me patience and empathy. (American Association of Caregiving Youth, 2006)

The majority of adult family caregivers work. Research shows the effects of family caregiving on the employed caregiver, the workplace, and the employer. Productivity declines as people worry about the one in their care or use work time for personal calls to schedule and coordinate care. They may arrive late or leave early, decrease their hours to part time, be unable to participate fully in advancement and learning opportunities, or quit their job altogether (Wagner, 2003). Education is the work life of young people. There is no reason to expect that the consequences of caregiving in the school work–life environment of an adolescent caregiver are much different from its consequences in the adult work environment. Both school-attending adolescents and working adults who are also family caregivers perform double duty.

Clearly, adolescent development involves many changes within the adolescent and in the dynamic ongoing interaction with the social environment. The findings of the National Youth Development and Information Center (2003) support the interrelationship between biological development and relationships. Maintenance of health and well-being in adolescents involves integrated physical and social development in the following categories: (a) physical activity, (b) competence and achievement, (c) self-definition, (d) creative expression, (e) positive social interactions with peers and adults, (f) structure and clear limits, and (g) meaningful participation (National Youth Development and Information Center, 2003).

U.S. RESEARCH ON ADOLESCENT CAREGIVERS

In the United States, studies on adolescent caregivers were undertaken beginning in the late 1990s. A brief discussion of some of these studies follows.

Life span developmental psychology involves multiple disciplines, including nursing, medicine, psychology, sociology, law, and biology (Papalia, Olds, & Feldman, 2007). Each discipline is driven by a different focus of research, with different goals, outcomes, and interventions. Because the research on adolescent caregiving has yielded varying results on the basis of samples that varied in size and demographics, the following discussion presents these studies in chronological order.

Two nurse practitioners, Gates and Lackey (1997), worked with families and caregiving youth. Their initial qualitative study used phenomenology, ethnography, and unstructured survey to demonstrate triangulation theory. Three data sets included 11 youth (11 to 19 years old; 3 boys, 8 girls) from seven English-speaking families. The persons requiring care ranged in age from 39 to 70 years. Caregiver roles changed depending on the severity of the care recipients' illness, the level of caregiving needed, and the availability of others to help. The most difficult tasks for the children were getting cigarettes, providing a urinal, or being there during times of pain instead of participating in a preferred activity (Gates & Lackey, 1997).

Understanding that development is multidimensional and trying to explain it in adolescent caregivers has challenges. Gates and Lackey (1997) discussed the process and complexities of creating a multidimensional picture of the young caregivers. For example, one 13-year-old informant described bathing and dressing her grandmother. When separately interviewed, the grandmother denied needing help with these activities. If the researchers had used only one source for information, the picture of the grandmother's need for assistance would be markedly different. Therefore, the researchers used a matrix model to combine various sources of information to portray a comprehensive view. The results produced three dichotomies faced by young caregivers: (a) the "hard yet gratifying" versus "challenging and burdensome" caregiving picture, (b) school as support versus school as a haven, and (c) focus on self versus focus on other person (Gates & Lackey, 1997).

Youth caregivers in the United States ascribe some benefits to their responsibilities as caregivers. Positive aspects of caregiving were reported by participants in the studies done by Gates and Lackey (1998), which found that youth learned new things and enjoyed the "I can do it myself" experiences. In all cases, school personnel were aware of the illness and caring situation. Parents and guardians sought help from school, church, and friends. Variability in school performance was found, with some individuals doing poorly and 1 student improving his grades (Gates & Lackey, 1998).

Beach's (1997) qualitative study of 20 adolescent caregivers, aged 14 to 18 years, reported varying responses to family caregiving for persons with Alzheimer's disease. Semistructured interviews and grounded theory methodology provided the format to learn about the subjective experiences of the young caregivers. Among the grouped responses listed as positive outcomes were increased sibling sharing and activity, increased empathy for older adults, significant mother–adolescent bonding, and discernment in peer relationship selection and maintenance. The group was mostly female (55%), Caucasian, and high school educated. The average age of the care receivers was 69 years, and the majority coresided. Humor as a coping skill yielded increased bonding among family members. Some distant relationships became closer as visits increased in frequency. One student learned to cultivate patience (Beach, 1997).

When a parent cared for a relative, relied on their own children, and included them as trusted confidants, the children's feelings of self-worth increased. In addition, some youth experienced more empathy for the parent who was having a difficult time with the caregiving role. Another outcome was that the young person learned to select friends on the basis of shared values. They had to feel that friends would understand if their grandparent's behavior or personality changed during a visit. Learning to build relationships based on common values may serve these young persons well in their future (Beach, 1997).

Orel and Dupuy (2002) studied three multigeneration families and used grounded theory to examine data previously obtained. They then used follow-up interviews, expert input, and triangulation to arrive at their analysis of qualitative data from 6 Caucasian youths from three families in which at least one primary caregiver was assisting a parent with personal care. The afflicted parent had dementia. The authors reviewed several coping strategies that families used and ultimately grouped their findings into positive and negative ramifications for the grandchildren.

The positive aspects included "feelings of gratification and satisfaction, closer relationships with the grandparents, and learned coping skills for the future" (p. 196). Contrasting effects were "negative view of aging, auxiliary caregiver burden, distant relationship with grandparents, and reduction in peer relationships" (p. 196).

In life span development theory, development is believed to be multidirectional. Although no longitudinal studies have been done on the effects of adolescent caregiving on adult development, a few retrospective studies have begun to address the effects of early caregiving roles on adult development.

Retrospective research promotes understanding of adolescent caregiving issues. Lackey and Gates (2001) interviewed 51 adults who had cared for family members during their childhood. More than half of the participants assisted with personal care such as bathing, toileting, and dressing and also helped with medical care such as giving pills or shots. Participants expressed the belief that early caregiving helped in the development of feelings of respect and compassion for others along with increased understanding of chronic illnesses. In addition, family life, school, and time with friends were adversely affected during the young caregiving years. Of the responsibilities and tasks these adults undertook as young caregivers, the most difficult was personal care, and the most time-consuming was performing household chores (Lackey & Gates, 2001). Lackey and Gates suggested that "parents and health care providers need to pay attention to the effects of caregiving on selected areas of youngsters' lives—particularly school and family life" (Lackey & Gates, 2001, p. 326).

Other researchers have found that when a parent has multiple sclerosis, his or her children are at risk for psychological problems, although 85% of parents saw no effect of their illness on their children (DeJudicibus & McCabe, 2004). Parents with cancer were also "surprised that their teenagers kept their feelings from them during this time, as they were not fully aware of the stress and overwhelming feelings of sadness and fear their adolescent children were experiencing" (Davey & Davey, 2005, p. 8).

Shifren and Kachorek (2003) reported about mental health effects from 24 adults from five states who were caregiving before the age of

21 years. Specifically, they showed the effects of child and adolescent caregiving on the caregivers' adult mental health. Each young caregiver had provided some personal care such as bathing, dressing, or feeding a parent or adult relative. The average age of the participants in this study was 13 years at the time they provided caregiving. The authors concluded that an early onset of the caregiving experience does "not automatically lead to adult mental health problems" (Shifren & Kachorek, 2003, p. 343).

Francine Cournos, professor of clinical psychiatry at Columbia University, was a youth caregiver. During the United Hospital Fund young caregivers stakeholders' meeting in October 2003, she discussed her tortuous journey of caregiving and provided a written account of her experiences (Cournos, 2003). Potential disadvantages that Cournos identified include traumatic exposure; interference with age-appropriate development; feelings of deprivation, inferiority, loss, and grief; and higher rates of psychiatric illness such as conduct disorder, depression, and posttraumatic stress syndrome. Among the possible advantages of the young caregiving role, she included competence, loyalty, emotional closeness to the person, ambition, and acceptance of death (Cournos, 2003).

In addition to the variety of U.S. studies on adolescent caregivers, there has been much research on adolescent caregiving experiences in other countries. Below is a discussion of some of the important findings from these studies.

A GLOBAL PERSPECTIVE

The issue of young persons caring for family members is global. Researchers in developed countries other than the United States have documented that youth often have a critical role in providing care within their family unit. Since the early 1990s, British researchers have been the global leaders in the identification of the roles and the effects of caregiving on young persons who have family caring responsibilities (e.g., Dearden & Becker, 2000). Studies have reported that the average age of a young person who has family caregiving responsibilities is 12 years in England (Carers National Association, 1997) and 13 years in Australia (Carers Australia, 2001). The *Final Report of the Young Carers Research Project* was published by the Commonwealth of Australia in 2001 (Carers Australia, 2001). It documents that young caregivers are "a significant, vulnerable, and disadvantaged group" who, when they are from minority populations, face a double disadvantage (p. 16).

Youth caregivers in the United Kingdom often experience bullying at school, with 70% reporting bullying at least once during their time as a caregiver (Princess Royal Trust for Carers, 1999). The deleterious effects of bullying create one of the most common needs for assistance. Among the reasons for bullying are that caregivers may have an unkempt appearance, be oversensitive or withdrawn, have minimal social skills, find it hard to develop friendships, be overly mature, or be ostracized because of family situations (Crabtree & Warner, 1999). In addition, shame may play a role both in children becoming the target of bullies and in the aftermath of having been bullied (Princess Royal Trust for Carers, 1999).

According to British, Irish, and Australian researchers, the impact of caregiving on youth are similar to the negative effects of caregiving on an adult. A young person may incur physical harm, particularly to the back, from limited sleep, carrying, lifting, and other physical demands (Carers Australia, 2001; Hill, 1999). When home responsibilities take priority over school and social activities, youth may experience isolation (Aldridge & Becker, 1993; Frank, 1995). A 2003 report from Wales determined that caregiving teens are "doubly disadvantaged" because they have limited financial resources and less time for socialization (Thomas et al. 2003, p. 40).

The Thomas et al. (2003) study reported that students understand the importance of education and its necessity for their future employment. Two teens left school because of the demands of their caregiving responsibilities but were anxious to return when they could. "Young carers frequently miss school because of their caring responsibilities; they have no time to complete homework, feel worried and distracted when they are at school, and experience limited connectedness with their school community" (p. 12). A 14-year-old girl claimed that she worried mainly "about the future, like if I don't go to school and don't pass my exams, how am I going to support my mum and my family, and that is my big worry" (p. 14).

Furthermore, long-term effects of caregiving by young persons include stress; depression; restricted social, educational, and career opportunities;

impaired psychosocial development; difficulty in transitioning to adulthood; and diminished opportunity for the future (Aldridge & Becker, 1993; Dearden & Becker, 2000; Frank, Tatum, & Tucker, 1999). In addition, emotional aspects of caregiving such as fear and worry can take a toll. Youth caregivers claim feelings of anger, resentment, exhaustion, and isolation (Frank, 1995; Thomas et al. 2003).

In addition to the adverse effects confronting youth caregivers around the world, there are positive aspects of caregiving. As in any challenging situation, young caregivers can benefit from the experience. During a focus group discussion, an Australian young person saw the aspect of role identification as a caregiver as positive empowerment and recognition: "Being called a young carer gives me identity in my role, what I do at home, not just to speak out to other people, but also in myself . . . to find that identity is amazing and was good" (Carers Australia, 2001, p. 20). Thomas et al. (2003) reported that some young people valued the caregiver experience because they perceived that it would prepare them for the future. They developed family closeness, and one boy felt prepared for college and his future.

It is clear from both U.S. research and international research that despite variations in demographics for adolescent caregivers, two contexts—school and home—are important. Less time at school and more time at home affect young caregivers' development. The first large study in the United States that looked at these contexts was the What Works Survey in Palm Beach County, Florida (B. Miller et al., 2003), which focused on the effects of adolescent caregiving on learning and academic performance. The information relative to family health situations and youth from the initial What Works Survey is limited; nevertheless, it was an important initial step.

THE WHAT WORKS SURVEY

The What Works Survey, conducted in 2002, was the first in the United States to query a large number of students about family health issues to learn whether health conditions, external to the education system, were a barrier to learning. The survey asked students if "they help someone needing special medical care in their home or close by." More than 12,681 students in 54 schools in Grades 6 to 12 participated in the survey. Of these, 6,210 students indicated that that they helped with care (Miller et al., 2003; Siskowski, 2003). In May 2003, 1,546 students in 14 private schools in Grades 4 through 12 took an amended version of the survey (Siskowski, 2004). More recently (April 2006), 1,895 middle and high school students in Largo, Florida, took an abbreviated form of the What Works Survey that focused specifically on the Family Health section (Siskowski, 2006c).

The What Works Survey Family Health section asks four basic questions: (a) Are there persons with special medical needs living in the homes of students or close by? (b) If so, do students feel that their family health situation hinders their ability to learn? (c) Are students helping with the provision of care? (d) If so, do students feel that participation in care affects their academic performance?

Students who completed the Family Health section indicated that they participated in care. The final survey question asked, "How does helping this person affect your academic performance in school?" Participants could choose from among the following answers: "I miss school/after school activities"; "I do not complete homework assignments"; "It interrupts my thinking and/or time studying"; "I have experienced more than one of the previous choices"; and "It has no affect on my performance at school."

Palm Beach County Public School Student Responses

Of the 12,681 students who began completing the largest survey (B. Miller et al., 2003; Siskowski, 2003), 11,029 answered Question 86, the final question in Section III before the Family Health section, and had the choice to stop or to continue the survey if it pertained to their situation. Three of 5 students (6,714, or 60.9%) continued the survey, thus indicating that there was someone in need of special medical care living with them or close by.

Similar to the entire student population of Palm Beach County, there were essentially an equal number of public school boys (49.8%) and girls (50.2%) among the students who identified their gender on the answer sheet. For unknown reasons, 9.1% of all the student survey participants did not identify themselves by gender. Of the 6,089 students who did and who answered the Family Health section, the split became uneven, with 3,399 boys (55.8%) and 2,690 girls (44.2%). Of these students, 2,326 either agreed or strongly agreed that living with the person in need of special medical care hindered their learning. Among these respondents, 57.2% were boys. The divide continued with the 5,612 students who identified themselves by gender and participated in care. Of these respondents, there were 3,159 boys (56.3%) and 2,453 girls (43.7%). Once again, boys outnumbered the girls (60% vs. 40%) in responding that participation in care adversely affected their academic performance. With both family health questions, the response differences between boys and girls was highly significant ($p < .001$).

The public school sample was culturally rich. Of the 11,029 students, 10,981 identified themselves by race. Of these, 6,678, or 60.8%, completed the Family Health section. Only the White non-Hispanic student population had a lower percentage of students responding to the Family Health section questions compared with their percentage of participation in the survey. This same group was significantly ($p < .001$) less affected than Blacks, who topped the list in every category when data within race were analyzed. When viewed from this perspective, 62.7% of Blacks had a person with special care needs in the family, 43.2% indicated this person hindered their learning, 94.3% participated in care, and 71.9% responded that their participation affected their academic performance.

What Works in Private Schools

The intent of the What Works project was to survey both public and private schools. With varying information needs among the public and private sectors, an amended private school survey followed the public school survey. There were 1,546 private school students in Grades 4 to 12 who took the private school version of the What Works Survey in May 2003.

Directions to stop or to continue the survey throughout the Family Health section remained constant. Thus, it was possible to use the same process that was used for the public school respondents to glean additional information about the prevalence of family health situations and student participation in care from the private school population.

Of the private school students participating in the survey, 656 answered the Family Health section. Of all students who began completing the survey, 42% had persons needing special medical care living with them or close by. On the basis of the same analytical process for both public and private school respondents, of the 1,546 students who began the survey, 1,476 students confronted the directions to stop or to continue the survey if they met the criteria and thus formed the analysis baseline. The overall private school prevalence for family health situations was 44.4%. The private school survey used a 4-point instead of a 5-point Likert scale for responses to questions assessing the effects on learning when a family health situation existed. Therefore, these answers are not fully comparable (Siskowski, 2003).

In light of the Palm Beach County data, the national study, and anecdotal information, school administrators of two schools in Largo, Florida (Pinellas County), opted to use an abbreviated form of the What Works Survey and focus only on the Family Health section. A summary of the primary results of all three surveys is in Table 2.1.

When there is a family health situation, the majority of students (89.9%) reported providing hands-on help regardless of any other ethnic or grade factor. In all cases, the majority of caregiving youth reported adverse effects. In contrast to national and international studies, the Palm Beach County private school results show that the percentage of boys who helped was significantly greater ($p < .001$) than girls (58.3% vs. 43.7%). Figure 2.1 provides a visual representation of these data.

Of special note is that the percentages among private school students who missed school or after school activities and who experienced more than one effect (15.8%) were greater than among Palm Beach County public school students (12.8%) in Grades 6 through 12. Unique in the Largo sample, the percentage of caregiving youth who experienced adverse effects increased with grade. Figure 2.2 shows these findings.

Table 2.1

Students With Family Health Situations, Caregiving Youth, and Those Reporting Adverse Effects From Caregiving From What Works Surveys

Category	2002 Palm Beach County Public Schools, Grades 6–12	2003 Palm Beach County Private Schools, Grades 6–12	2006 Largo Middle and Largo High Schools	Total
Family Health question baseline[a] (n)	9,799	835	1895	12,871
Answered Family Health section[a] (n)	5,860	417	569	7,028
Prevalence of family health situations (%)	59.8	49.9	30.0	54.6
Caregiving youth[a] (n)	5,407	374	534	6,315
Participated in caregiving (%)	92.3	83.2	93.8	89.9
Reported adverse effects (%)	63.7	55.1	52.8	57.2

Note. 1,585 students in the public school survey did not identify themselves by grade, and 329 private school students did not identify themselves by grade. Data extracted by C. Siskowski from original data files of What Works Survey in Palm Beach County Public Schools, modified What Works Survey in Private Schools, and Abbreviated What Works Survey in Largo Schools. Although the whole survey content changed, the Family Health questions on all surveys remained constant.
[a]Only those identified by grade.

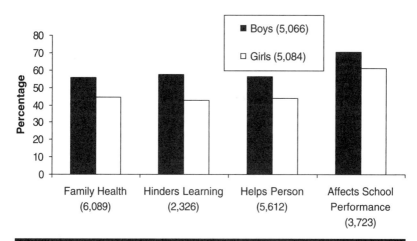

Figure 2.1

The What Works Survey results from Palm Beach County, Florida public schools. Note that 879 students did not identify themselves by gender. Data are from Siskowski (2003). Family Health = respondent indicated he or she had a health situation in the family possibly requiring caregiving.

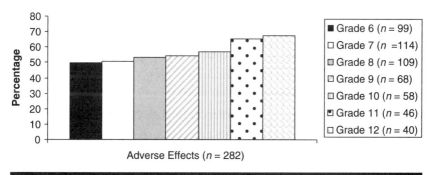

Figure 2.2

Among 1,895 Largo, Florida, middle school and Largo high school students who participated in the abbreviated What Works Survey, 569 were caregiving youth, and of these, 282 experienced adverse effects. The percentage of students with adverse effects increased with each grade. Data are from Siskowski (2006b).

SUMMARY AND CONCLUSION

It is clear from the findings of the What Works Survey that development is affected by the school and home contexts; students reported increased time at home and decreased time at school. The survey shows that adolescent development is affected by the caregiving role, with varying effects on learning and academic performance. Findings also show gender differences in the effects of caregiving for a relative on learning and academic performance (congruent with reported gender differences in caregiving in the gerontology literature; Yee & Schulz, 2000). Adolescent boys reported that providing care to a relative adversely affected their school performance more than did adolescent girls. Black adolescents reported providing more care to a relative and had poorer school performance because of such caregiving than White adolescents. With regard to providing more care than Whites, there is evidence for the same result in older adult caregiving samples comparing Black and White caregivers (Mak, 2005).

Many adolescent caregivers, especially those who are disadvantaged by economic inadequacies and limited adult support, incur adverse effects from their caregiving responsibilities. National and international reports are consistent in reporting these effects. As mentioned in chapter 1 of this volume, impoverished environments may include not only a lack of finances but support. It is also clear that there is the opportunity for youth caregivers to learn life skills and develop value systems through their caregiving experiences that will assist them in later life. The recognition and support needed by caregiving youth can come from within healthy family units that work as a team to manage and address a family health situation.

In their discussion of future work, Shifren and Kachorek (2003) expressed concern that the work of youth caregivers will be taken for granted and considered an integral component of care delivery in the United States. If this occurs, a diminished need for the development of social support networks would result, and the role of the care recipients as parents and the importance of family would be compromised.

Ways to Help Adolescent Caregivers

Through caregiving, adolescents can learn valuable life skills. Barkley (2003) discussed using the power of real-life experiences as an educational tool. A life experience or life event is a multisensory experience involving sight, hearing, and touch. A person uses both basic and complex skills when participating in life events. Events are relevant to the student: An event is real, attached to emotion. Barkley stated, "Students are engaged when something has real meaning. Something is at stake; it counts" (p. 132). Students who are caregivers are engaged at two levels. First, they are already part of a life event in which one person is relying on another for help in making it through the day. Second, they are engaged because they want to do a good job; this is made even more challenging by the fact that it is likely that they have received little formal training or recognition.

Other researchers have looked at the needs of youth caregivers. Gates and Lackey (1998) identified three groups of needs expressed by caregiving youth: (a) time for themselves and their personal needs, (b) needs related to the adult with cancer, and (c) relationship needs with family and others. Gates and Lackey stated that although "school time was protected, their time for playing, studying, and private pursuits were most affected" (p. 14).

Gates and Lackey (1998) also reported that youth want information: "Youngsters express anger when they are not told that the diagnosis is cancer" (p. 13). Additional findings included that school was respite and that the caring interfered with having friends over, playing with friends, and homework. "Youngsters express fear regarding something happening to the adult, doing something wrong, or being left alone. Often the youngsters described feeling fatigued" (p. 13). The youngsters did not want to talk with others about their caregiving activities. They prayed, read their Bibles, thought positively, and just tried to deal with the situation. When there were multiple siblings, the oldest assumed most of the responsibility (Gates & Lackey, 1998).

Adolescent caregivers want more information. For example, adolescents realize they are part of the health care team. They want to learn specifics about medical conditions and what to expect as a consequence of an illness. In addition, they want to know life skills, including communication techniques and problem solving. Worsham and Crawford (2005) noted that caregiving youth want "safe people" with whom to talk, reciprocal relationships, and a supportive environment. They encouraged professionals to gain individual information from youth, respond to them in a timely way, be sensitive to the complexities of their development versus their caregiving role, teach life skills, and help caregiving families discern the controllable and noncontrollable contributing factors to stress (Worsham & Crawford, 2005).

There is a compelling need for the development of and access to support services for youth caregivers. The first U.S. Caregiving Youth Project began as a pilot in Boca Raton, Florida, in early September 2006 to develop a school-based support model. It began with a Web-based survey for all students with parental consent. These survey data were used for baseline identification and evaluation. Project enrollees received multiple interventions: in-school counseling, education, in-home evaluation with linkages to existing resources, sponsored individual and family activities, an overnight camp, and respite. By the 2007–2008 academic year, the Caregiving Youth Project had expanded to three middle schools in Southern Palm Beach County. In another region of Palm Beach County, caregiving eighth-grade students who were unlikely to access caregiving support services were identified by using basic questions of the same Web-based survey. After 3 years, school dropout rates for caregiving students with intervention and support will be compared with those without intervention and support.

The American Association of Caregiving Youth (AACY; see http://www.aacy.org) lists Web resources and provides a toll-free number (800-725-2512). The AACY Web site has portals for preteens, teens, families, and professionals. AACY is formally organized under the auspices of Volunteers for the Homebound and Family Caregivers, a nonprofit Florida corporation. Assistance from the Princess Royal Trust for Carers in the United Kingdom, the Australia Carers, and national disease-specific organizations in the United States augment the development and progress of needed resources for caregiving youth. This approach to solutions recognizes the need for collaboration among many disciplines, along with systems and multidisciplinary integration.

DIRECTIONS FOR FUTURE RESEARCH

The findings of various studies compel additional research to promote better understanding of the extent to which culturally diverse groups of students engage in caregiving roles and the range of caregiving activities that affect their lives. Longitudinal studies to document the long-term effects of caregiving experiences on youth caregivers are critical to the future well-being of adolescents and caregiving families in the United States. It is important to understand how differences among various familial relationships as well as disease-specific and aging-related caregiving situations affect children. Whether the adolescent is the primary or secondary caregiver, there is opportunity to learn about and prevent adverse health consequences that may result from caregiving.

In late September 2006, the National Alliance for Caregiving and the National Multiple Sclerosis Society hosted its second national conference in Washington, DC, to address the issues and policies that surround caregiving youth. Although work has begun, there is much yet to do in all arenas. Although the United States is a decade behind the United Kingdom, now is the time for the development of both short- and long-term support of caregiving adolescents and their families. Then these dual-role students will have the opportunity to become healthy, educated, and productive citizens of tomorrow.

REFERENCES

Aldridge, J., & Becker, S. (1993). *Children who care: Inside the world of young carers*. Leicestershire, England: Loughborough University, Young Carers Research Group.

American Association of Caregiving Youth. (2006). *George Snow scholarship winners*. Retrieved April 13, 2008, from http://www.aacy.org/teen/snow%20biography/biography.htm

American Association of Caregiving Youth. (n.d.). *Miriam from Nebraska*. Retrieved April 14, 2008, from http://www.aacy.org/publications/heroes2/slides/ScreenShot030.html

Barkley, S. (2003). Motivating students with live-event learning. *Kappa Delta Pi Record, 39*, 130–133.

Beach, D. L. (1997). Family caregiving: The positive impact on adolescent relationships. *The Gerontologist, 37,* 233–238.

Butler, R. (2001). *Old and poor in America.* New York: International Longevity Center—USA.

Carers Australia. (2001). *Young carers research project final report.* Canberra: Commonwealth of Australia, Department of Family and Community Services: Author.

Carers National Association. (1997). *In on the act?* London: Author.

Cournos, F. (2003, October). *The psychological impact of being a young caregiver.* Paper presented at a Young Caregivers meeting by the United Hospital Fund Foundation, New York.

Crabtree, H., & Warner, L. (1999). *Too much to take on: A report on young carers and bullying.* London: The Princess Royal Trust for Carers.

Davey, M., & Davey, A. (2005). Adolescents coping with non-terminal parental cancer. *The Prevention Researcher, 12*(4), 7–9.

Dearden, C., & Becker, S. (2000). *Growing up and caring: Vulnerability and transition to adulthood—Young carers' experiences.* Leicester, England: Youth Work Press.

DeJudicibus, M. A., & McCabe, M. P. (2004). The impact of parental multiple sclerosis on the adjustment of children and adolescents. *Adolescents, 39,* 551–569.

Dilworth-Anderson, P., Williams, S. W., & Cooper, T. (1999). Family caregiving to elderly African-Americans: Caregiving types and structures. *Journal of Gerontology: Social Sciences, 54*(B), 5237–5241.

Eccles, J. S. (2004). Schools, academic motivation, and stage–environment fit. In R. Lerner & L. Steinberg (Eds.), *Handbook of adolescent psychology* (pp. 125–153). New York: Wiley.

Erikson, E. H. (1968). *Identity: Youth and crisis.* New York: Norton.

Faulkner, R. A., & Davey, M. (2002). Children and adolescents of cancer patients: The impact of cancer on the family. *American Journal of Family Therapy, 30,* 63–72.

Federal Interagency Forum on Child and Family Statistics. (2000). *America's children: Key national indicators of well-being 2002.* Retrieved March 19, 2008, from http://www.childstats.gov/pdf/ac2000/body.pdf

Florida Department of Health. (2001). *Public health indicator reports, 1998–2000.* Tallahassee: Author.

Frank, J. (1995). *Couldn't care more: A study of young carers and their needs.* London: The Children's Society.

Frank, J., Tatum, C., & Tucker, S. (1999). *On small shoulders: Learning from the experiences of former young carers.* London: The Children's Society.

Gates, M. F., & Lackey, N. R. (1997). Combining the analyses of three qualitative data sets in studying young caregivers. *Journal of Advanced Nursing, 26,* 664–671.

Gates, M. F., & Lackey, N. R. (1998). Youngsters caring for adults with cancer. *Image: The Journal of Nursing Scholarship, 30*, 11–15.

Goodnow, J. J. (1988). Children's household work: Its nature and functions. *Psychological Bulletin, 103*, 5–26.

Hill, S. (1999). The physical effects of caring on children. *Journal of Young Carers Work, 3*, 6–7.

Kiecolt-Glaser, J. K., Preacher, K. J., MacCallum, R. C., Atkinson, C., Malarkey, W. B., & Glaser, R. (2003). Chronic stress and age-related increases in the proinflammatory cytokine IL-6. *Proceedings of the National Academy of Sciences, USA 100*(15), 9090–9095.

Knight, B. G., Silverstein, M., McCallum, T. J., & Fox, L. S. (2000). A sociocultural stress and coping model for mental health outcomes among African-American caregivers in Southern California. *Journal of Gerontology: Psychological Sciences, 55*(B), 142–50.

Lackey, N. R., & Gates, M. F. (2001). Adults' recollections of their experiences as young caregivers of family members with chronic physical illnesses. *Journal of Advanced Nursing, 34*, 320–328.

Lamorey, S. (1999). *Parentification of siblings of children with disability of chronic disease: Burdened children.* Thousand Oaks, CA: Sage.

Lifespan Respite Care Act of 2006, H.R. 3248, 109th Cong., Public Law No. 109-442. (2006).

Mak, W. W. (2005). Integrative model of caregiving: How macro and micro factors affect caregivers of adults with severe and persistent mental illness. *American Journal of Ortho psychiatry, 75*, 40–53.

Miller, B., Bunker, M., & Kelley-Miller, G. (2003). *What works: What do students think? Final report.* West Palm Beach, FL: Palm Beach Atlantic University.

Miller, N. B., & Sammons, C. C. (1999). *Everybody's different.* Baltimore: Brookes.

National Alliance for Caregiving & American Association of Retired Persons. (2004). *Caregiving in the U.S.* Washington, DC: Author.

National Alliance for Caregiving & The United Hospital Fund. (2005). *Young caregivers in the U.S.* Washington, DC: Author.

National Center for Health Statistics. (2007). *Health, United States, 2007: With chartbook on trends in the health of Americans.* Retrieved April 13, 2008, from http://www.cdc.gov/nchs/data/hus/hus07.pdf#104

National Middle School Association. (2003). *Supporting students in their transition to middle school.* Retrieved April 13, 2003, from http://www.nmsa.org/news.transition.html

National Youth Development & Information Center. (2003). *Definitions of youth development.* Retrieved January 25, 2004, from http://www.nydic.org/nydic/devdef.html

Orel, N. A., & Dupuy, P. (2002). Grandchildren as auxiliary caregivers for grandparents with cognitive and/or physical limitations: Coping strategies and ramifications. *Child Study Journal, 32,* 193–213.

Papalia, D. E., Olds, S. W., & Feldman, R. D. (2007). *Human development.* Boston: McGraw-Hill.

Princess Royal Trust for Carers. (1999). *Too much to take on—A report on young carers and bullying.* London: Author.

Rizzo, V. M., & Kirkland, K. A. (2005). Adolescent reactions to parental cancer: Strategies for providing support. *The Prevention Researcher, 12*(4), 10–12.

Sahyoun, N. R., Pratt, L. A., Lentzner, H., Dey, A., & Robinson, K. N. (2001). *The changing profile of nursing home residents: 1985–1997.* Hyattsville, MD: National Center for Health Statistics.

Schulz, R., & Beach, S. R. (1999). Caregiving as a risk factor for mortality: the Caregiver Health Effects Study. *JAMA, 282,* 2215–2219.

Shifren, K. (2001). Early caregiving and adult depression: Good news for young caregivers. *The Gerontologist, 41,* 188–190.

Shifren, K., & Kachorek, L. V. (2003). Does early caregiving matter? The effects on young caregivers' adult mental health. *International Journal of Behavioral Development, 27,* 338–346.

Siskowski, C. (2003). *From their eyes . . . Family health situations influence students' learning and lives in Palm Beach County, Grades 6–12.* Retrieved May 1, 2006, from http://www.boca-respite.org/children.doc

Siskowski, C. T. (2004). Middle school student responses to family health questions: The effects of family caregiving on the education of middle school students with family health issues. *Dissertation Abstracts International.* (UMI No. 3142225)

Siskowski, C. (2006a). *Caregiving youth in Largo middle and high schools, Largo, Florida.* Retrieved December 26, 2007, from http://aacy.org/publications/publications.htm

Siskowski, C. (2006b). *Final report: Largo middle and high schools, Largo, Florida.* Retrieved April 14, 2008, from www.aacy.org/publications/final%20report%20/largo.doc

Siskowski, C. (2006c). Young caregivers: Effect of family health situations on school performance. *Journal of School Nursing, 22,* 163–169.

Thomas, N., Stainton, T., Jackson, S., Cheung, W. Y., Doubtfire, S., & Webb, A. (2003). "Your friends don't understand": Invisibility and unmet need in the lives of "young carers." *Child and Family Social Work, 8,* 35–46.

U.S. Census Bureau. (2001). *Profiles of general demographic characteristics of population, 2000.* Retrieved November 11, 2003, from http://www.census.gov/prod/2003pubs/c2kbr-29.pdf

U.S. Department of Health and Human Services. (1998). *Informal caregiving: Compassion in action.* Washington, DC: Author.

U.S. Department of Health and Human Services. (2004). *About NFCSP.* Retrieved March 11, 2004, from http://www.aoa.gov/prof/aoaprog/caregiver/overview/ overview_caregiver.asp

U.S. Department of Labor. (2006, August). *National compensation survey: Employee benefits in private industry in the United States.* Retrieved April 13, 2008, from http://www.bls.gov/ncs/ebs/sp/ ebsm0004.pdf

Wagner, D. L. (2003). *Workplace programs for family caregivers: Good business and good practice.* Retrieved June 5, 2004, from http://www.caregiver.org/ caregiver/jsp/content_node.jsp?nodeid=953

Wang, Q. (2005). *Disability and American families: 2000* (CENSR-23). Retrieved March 19, 2008, from http://www.census.gov/prod/2005pubs/censr-23.pdf

Williams, S. W. (2002). Systems of social support in families who care for dependent African American elders. *The Gerontologist, 42,* 224–226.

Worsham, N. L., & Crawford, E. K. (2005). Parental illness and adolescent development. *The Prevention Researcher, 12*(4), 3–6.

Yee, J. L., & Schulz, R. (2000). Gender differences in psychiatric morbidity among family caregivers: A review and analysis. *The Gerontologist, 40,* 147–164.

3

Emerging and Young Adulthood and Caregiving

Mary Dellmann-Jenkins and Maureen Blankemeyer

According to life span development theory, a person's history affects his or her development (Baltes, Lindenberger, & Staudinger, 1998). Improvements in technology, medicine, and nutrition that have led to longer lives are a part of that history (Papalia, Olds, & Feldman, 2007). As discussed previously in this book, longer lives are also associated with increased chances for illness (Verbrugge, 1989). Given older adults' desire to remain in their homes as long as possible, the results of recent analyses depicting families as "the backbone of long-term care provision" in the United States are not surprising (Wolff & Kasper, 2006, p. 351). However, the recent trend of emerging adults (ages 18 to 25 years) and young adults (ages 26 to 40 years) contributing to the family-based long-term care workforce in the United States may be surprising to some because only a few research papers have been published on this caregiving topic (Dellmann-Jenkins, Blankemeyer, & Pinkard, 2000, 2001; Dellmann-Jenkins & Brittain, 2003; Levine, Hunt, Halper, Hart, Lautz, & Gould, 2005; Shifren, 2001; Shifren & Kachorek, 2003).

National caregiving surveys indicate that between 17% and 28% of unpaid primary caregivers to disabled older adults living in the community are emerging and young adults (Levine et al., 2005; Wolff & Kasper, 2006). On the basis of on our research, for many young people the acquisition of the caregiver role to elderly relatives coincides with making critical personal, family life, and career development decisions. Our major findings also characterize these emerging and young adult children and grandchildren as displaying high levels of filial responsibility and frequently motivated by a sense of generational reciprocity to assume the caregiving role in order to help out their middle-aged parents.

This chapter reviews the major developmental tasks of emerging and young adulthood and then outlines how the responsibilities and challenges of caring for older family members may affect the successful accomplishment of these tasks. This chapter also presents our findings on young caregivers' sense of filial responsibility toward elderly relatives and actual caregiving behaviors. Although the minority of participants in our research were emerging adults (40% in the 2000 study and 32% in the 2003 study), these data are provided separately from the data on young adults when appropriate. In addition, recommendations are made on informal and formal support services that may enhance the caregiving role of emerging and young adults while assisting them with issues typical to their life stages. The chapter closes with several recommendations for future research.

EMERGING AND YOUNG ADULTHOOD

The years between 18 and 40, often referred to as *early adulthood* or *young adulthood* (e.g., Santrock, 2007), are marked by profound changes and life-shaping decisions (Schaie & Willis, 2002). People in this age range typically experience the following developmental processes: (a) differentiation from parents and others, (b) formation of intimate relationships, and (c) establishment of economic independence (e.g., Erikson, 1968). These tasks have been identified as crucial for setting the foundation for development across the remainder of the life span. Although the tasks traditionally have been associated with young adulthood, it is important to recognize their role within a recently conceived developmental period, *emerging adulthood*, which extends from the ages 18 to 25 years (Arnett, 2000). Because emerging adulthood is a relatively new concept, a description of this period is provided in the following section. For the present purposes, emerging adulthood refers to those aged 18 to 25 years, and young adulthood includes 26- to 40-year-olds. This is not to imply that chronological age serves as a rigid boundary that differentiates various stages along the developmental trajectory. Rather, the age ranges are intended to serve as general markers for when developmental processes typically occur.

Emerging Adulthood

Arnett (2000) coined the term *emerging adulthood* to depict the unique developmental period that extends from 18 to 25 years. The term *emerging* is used to capture the fact that people of this age often are at an unsettled point in their lives where they are exploring significant life possibilities (e.g., career, partner) that will set the foundation for a stable life structure. Emerging adulthood ushers in a new independence for the young person, typically beginning at age 18 when most Americans complete high school and move out of their parents' home. Until relatively recently, this time of life was dense with developmental milestones typically associated with adulthood, such as completion of education, marriage, parenthood, and the establishment of a career. However, these indicators of adult status now occur later on average than they did 50 years ago. For example, young people in the United States increasingly are seeking postsecondary education. Currently, 23% of women and 25% of men have obtained a bachelor's degree or higher (U.S. Census Bureau, 2005). This, in turn, has resulted in an increase in the age at which many young people enter the labor force full time. Marriages also occur at later ages than they did historically. In 1955, the median age at first marriage was 22.6 years for men and 20.2 years for women. In 2005, the median age at first marriage was 27.1 years for men and 25.8 years for women (U.S. Census Bureau, 2006). Americans are not only marrying later but are also having children later (Azar, 2003). Thus, the path from adolescence to adulthood is now lengthier than it used to be.

Because many 18- to-25-year-olds have not yet reached the developmental milestones of adulthood, Arnett (2000) distinguished this period as distinct from young adulthood. Emerging adulthood also is distinct from adolescence because 18- to-25-year-olds generally are more independent from their parents than are adolescents, and their lives are much more heterogeneous than those of adolescents (Arnett & Tanner, 2006). These young people's trajectories through work, school, and romantic relation-ships vary considerably, with some choosing to marry, others remaining single, many enrolling in college, others opting for employment instead, and still others combining both school and employment. Unlike the heterogeneity of emerging adulthood, there is little demographic variation among adolescents, most of whom live with their parents and are single. Another important reason why Arnett (2000) distinguished emerging adulthood as a unique developmental period is that 18- to 25-year-olds perceive themselves as neither adolescents nor adults.

As young people exit adolescence, they acquire new traits, including an improved ability to understand others' perspectives and increased consid-eration for others (Arnett, 2004). These qualities may help explain why some emerging and young adults take on the role of caregiver to an older relative. Because a key principle of lifespan development is that develop-ment is multidimensional, we address a number of aspects of development in this chapter. Following are descriptions of the developmental processes that emerging and young adults experience. The ways in which these tasks are affected by the caregiving role also are discussed.

Developmental Processes During Emerging and Young Adulthood

Differentiation From the Family of Origin

The task of *differentiation*, or *emancipation*, from the family of origin involves establishing independent yet harmonious relationships with one's parents and siblings. Those who successfully differentiate themselves from their family of origin are able to cope effectively with being apart from their parents (Scharf, Mayseless, & Kivenson-Baron, 2004) and can make independent, competent decisions (Arnett, 2001). Accomplishment of this task is crucial in the development of a unique personal identity for the young person and in his or her ability to successfully establish true inti-macy with dating and marriage partners (Erikson, 1980). It is important to note that differentiation does not imply disengagement from the fam-ily of origin. Fuligni and Pedersen (2002) reported that young people's sense of obligation to support and assist their families increases significantly in the 3 years after they graduate from high school.

The process of differentiation usually begins with the young person moving from the family home. Current statistics indicate that most individuals (at least two thirds) are living independently by their mid-20s (White, 1994); therefore, the task of differentiation is more likely to commence in emerging adulthood than in young adulthood. However, analyses of recent cohorts of 18- to 25-year-olds indicate that nearly one half return home at least briefly (Goldscheider & Goldscheider, 1999; Ward & Spitze, 2007). The process of differentiation for some individuals may extend into their 30s (young adulthood years).

Although establishing an independent residence is a crucial component of differentiation, more than one half (57%) of the young filial caregivers in our research shared a household with the older care recipient (Dellmann-Jenkins et al., 2001). The majority of young caregivers (82%) reported positive outcomes from the living arrangement, including developing a closer relationship with the care recipient because of increased time spent together, seeing extended family members more frequently because of their visits to the care recipient, and instrumental assistance from the care recipient (e.g., housing, food, or assistance with child care). In some instances (18%), the 18- to 40-year-olds reported receiving financial assistance from the older care recipient. In all of these cases, the young caregivers receiving such assistance from the older care recipient were unemployed or underemployed and living with the older family member.

Establishing Intimate Relationships

Emancipation from the family of origin lays the foundation for successful accomplishment of the second developmental process: the establishment of close emotional relationships with friends and dating partners, spouses, and children (e.g., Camp & Ganong, 1997; Erikson, 1980).

Friendships and dating. Friendships that involve mutual trust, respect, understanding, and acceptance can be important buffers against the effects of stress experienced by caregivers during emerging and young adulthood.

During these developmental periods, individuals establish more affiliative bonds and have a wider range of acquaintances than at any other stage (Carstensen, 1992). This may help explain why decreased depressive symptoms and increased self-esteem are apparent beginning in emerging adulthood (Schulenberg, Bryant, & O'Malley, 2004). However, this time of improved psychological well-being may not characterize those who do not engage in their friendship networks because of time constraints resulting from the filial caregiver role. The emerging and young adults in our research reported that time normally spent with friends had been replaced with performing caregiving responsibilities (Dellmann-Jenkins et al., 2001). All of our participants were providing some type of daily assistance to an older relative and spending at least 3 hours per day in the caregiving role (Dellmann-Jenkins et al., 2000). Thus, it is not surprising that many (47%) reported that time for social activities had been hindered by their caregiving role. A 20-year-old granddaughter disclosed, "I sometimes get mad because I think I am doing too much for my grandpa and I don't have a life of my own . . . then I feel selfish for having such thoughts."[1]

Dating relationships also are affected by the filial caregiving role. The single participants in our research were asked about their dating lives and ability to establish and maintain romantic relationships. The majority of them (68%) replied that the amount of time given to their caregiving responsibilities made this aspect of their lives very difficult (Dellmann-Jenkins et al., 2001). Single young men were as verbal as their female counterparts regarding this issue. For example, a 26-year-old man who was taking care of his 86-year-old grandfather stated, "My social life is almost dead! Dating seems very limited because I hardly have time for myself." A common concern for the unmarried participants focused on whether to ask a partner to commit to such an involved and unpredictable family relationship.

Marriage. Erikson (1982) regarded marriage as a crucial task of young adulthood. Many young people today are postponing this task until the beginning of the young adult years instead of accomplishing it during

---

[1] All quotes from caregivers throughout this chapter are from Dellmann-Jenkins et al. (2000, pp. 181–184).

the emerging adult years, as used to be the case (U.S. Census Bureau, 2006). Some young people prefer to obtain a college education before marrying, some are deterred by the high divorce rate in our society, and some prefer to cohabit rather than marry. All of these factors contribute to the societal trend of young people marrying at later ages. In addition, as discussed above, the caregiver role hindered the dating relationships of most of the single participants in our research, suggesting that they may have postponed marriage because of their filial responsibilities.

The caregiving role affects not only when an individual marries but also the marital relationships of emerging and young adults. In our research, when married participants were asked about how their caregiving role had affected their marital relationship, only 22% reported that their spouses were supportive (Dellmann-Jenkins et al., 2001). The majority of the married respondents (83%) reported that time spent with their partner had decreased, the relationship had been negatively affected as a result of the caregiving responsibilities, or both. One 26-year-old man who had cared for his father stated, "I don't think we would have felt as much stress as we did if we hadn't just recently been married." A 33-year-old woman revealed that intimate times were awkward because of her mother's presence in the home. Another reported that she could not spend enough time with her spouse because they took separate shifts caring for her grandmother. A 26-year-old who was assisting her grandparents stated,

> I would like to go camping with my husband once in a while, but I can't just get up and go away because of taking care of my grandparents. Even though they have the medical alert, I am afraid that they won't use it if something goes wrong.

Other young caregivers reported much more stress in their relationships. One granddaughter disclosed, "It was very hard on my marriage. My husband and I separated for a while. He was so angry, he refused to go to grandfather's funeral." In our research, the emerging and young adults did not differ in marital strain resulting from the caregiving role.

Parenthood. It is most often during the young adult years that the decision is made to become a parent or remain childless. Although just over one half of births in the United States are to women in their 20s, birth rates to women in their 30s and older have increased substantially (Martin et al., 2003). Along with providing an enhanced sense of self-worth, satisfaction, and a feeling of adult status, the introduction of the first child into the family signals a series of significant lifestyle changes and challenges for new parents, such as added financial strain (Lino, 2002), forgone wages and other opportunity costs (Crittenden, 2001), and marital strain (Twenge, Campbell, & Foster, 2003).

In our research, the emerging and young adults' parenting role appeared to be affected by their caregiving role, and vice versa. Nearly one fourth (22%) of these young caregivers with children under age 18 reported positive outcomes specifically related to their children's relationship with the older care recipient. When asked the question, "What do you find most satisfying or rewarding about assisting your elderly family member?" a 28-year-old woman who was caring for her 83-year-old grandmother-in-law replied, "Her relationship with my daughter." Other mothers mentioned that the care recipient had been beneficial to them by providing child care from time to time. Alternatively, in at least one case, the children facilitated the older relative's care. According to a single parent of three young children, "The children help me with grandma. We all do it together. Grandma interacts better with the children because she trusts them. She will take her medicine for my daughter, but not for me." In contrast, a 26-year-old woman explained, "My 2-year-old son often gets on my grandparents' nerves. They can't stand the noise. When I take them to appointments, I have to arrange for a sitter to care for my son."

Economic Independence

In addition to differentiating themselves from their families of origin and establishing intimate relationships, emerging adults are typically exploring ways to become financially independent. Young adults, however, generally are more settled into their jobs than emerging adults. Emerging adults are considering what kind of work they are good at and try out different jobs, or those in college explore different majors in preparation for their intended occupation. Some young people enter directly into the labor force, and others pursue postsecondary education first as a means to eventual financial autonomy. Educational attainment is considered to be the event most likely to influence the timing of later significant life events, such as work, marriage, and parenting (Teachman & Paasch, 1998). In 1999, 45% of emerging adults were enrolled in college (Barton, 2002). Often, young people are simultaneously enrolled in college while also employed in the labor force. In 2001, nearly 43% of college freshmen who were enrolled full time were in the labor force (U.S. Department of Labor, 2002, cited in Arnett & Tanner, 2006).

Among the young caregivers in our research, 18% were juggling caregiving along with the responsibilities of being a college student. All of these young people reported that they had "less time to study" and "had to miss classes" as a result of their elder caregiver roles.

Typical college students today experience more stress and depression than in the past (Sax, Lindholm, Astin, Korn, & Mahoney, 2002), and those who concurrently are in the caregiving role may be at heightened risk for mental health problems. However, research thus far suggests that early caregiving does not lead to poor mental health for many young caregivers (Shifren & Kachorek, 2003). In addition, because higher education is associated with higher income, young caregivers who must forgo or postpone an education because of their filial responsibilities may be limiting their economic potential when they acquire the caregiver role.

Regardless of the path taken toward financial independence, taking on the new role of full-time employee can be a significant source of both satisfaction and stress when added to the other developmental tasks and the filial caregiving responsibilities. Those who are employed are more satisfied with their lives and are physically healthier than those who are unemployed (Barnett & Marshall, 1992a, 1992b). However, young employees report higher negative spillover than others do (Moen, 1999). They are more likely to experience stress in their family that spills over and affects their work, and vice versa. These negative spillover effects were apparent in our research. More than one fourth (26%) of the emerging and young adults perceived that their career goals had been negatively affected as a result of their caregiving roles. A 27-year-old woman who was caring for an elderly parent commented, "I was building a career when my mother became ill. I will never attain the goals that I had set for my career." Others (15%) believed that they missed the opportunity for job promotions as a result of their caregiving role. One 26-year-old who had to quit his job to care for his 89-year-old grandfather candidly stated, "I wish I knew how long I will have to put my career on hold in order to do this. He could live to be 100 years old. Where will I be then?" Furthermore, 22% stated that they had either quit a job at one point in their role as caregiver or were not working at the time of the interview because of their caregiving responsibilities.

A large portion of both the emerging adults and the young adults in our research indicated that their caregiving responsibilities had negatively affected their ability to relocate, which then resulted in limited employment opportunities (Dellmann-Jenkins et al., 2000). As a 27-year-old woman who was caring for her mother revealed, "I am unable to relocate to . . . a larger city where I could get a better job." A 25-year-old female caregiver similarly responded, "I was offered a better position with the company that I currently work for, but I was unable to relocate." Other young caregivers indicated that their spouses had either turned down a better job or were not able to move closer to their present work site because of the need to live near the care recipient. A 26-year-old woman who was caring for both of her grandparents commented,

> My husband would like to move closer to his job, but that would not work because I am caring for my grandparents. And one time he was offered a job out-of-state, but we can't even think about that as long as I am caring for my grandparents.

Nearly one half (48%) of the employed young caregivers reported that their workplace attendance had been negatively affected as a result of their caregiving responsibilities. Yet, most of the young workers said that they could not afford to miss work: "I have just started a new job and I can't miss work. There are times when I need to, but I just can't." Overall, the emerging adults and young adults did not differ in work-related strain resulting from their caregiving roles (Dellmann-Jenkins et al., 2001).

Emerging and young adult caregivers are facing the tasks of differentiation, establishing family and other intimate relationships, and building their economic independence while assuming the role of caregiver. Our research indicated that the caregiving role affected these developmental processes. Many of our respondents were not living independently from the care recipient, and although many reported positive outcomes from this arrangement, their social and family relationships were negatively affected and their career path was often hindered by their filial responsibilities. These results were found for both emerging and young adults in our research.

EMERGING AND YOUNG ADULTS' SENSE OF FILIAL RESPONSIBILITY TOWARD OLDER FAMILY MEMBERS

Filial responsibility refers to the idea of children being willing to care for aging parents and relatives without economic incentive (Wolfsen, Hanfield-Jones, Glass, McClaren, & Keyserlingk, 1993). The recent trend of emerging adults and young adults who are providing daily care to older family members—often living with the care recipient to avoid nursing home placement—challenges an earlier conception of filial roles in these developmental periods. Blenkner's (1965) classic model depicts (a) the development of filial responsibility as a feature unique to the middle years of adulthood and (b) emerging and young adulthood as characterized by filial immaturity, where a sense of duty or willingness to support elderly relatives has yet to develop. Our research on young people in caregiving roles to older family members led to an alternative perspective for the development of filial responsibility: one that focuses more on the influence of the family environment and less on the impact of chronological age in determining whether one assumes filial responsibility. Therefore, our research is more consistent with Baltes's (1987) life span model than with Blenkner's age-related model of filial responsibility. Baltes proposed that development in adulthood is (a) multicausal in nature, (b) primarily the result of the social context and historic time, and (c) not the result of the mere passage of time. Application of Baltes's view of adult development to current family trends led to two underlying assumptions that guided our research on young caregivers:

1. Increased chronological age, in itself, does not result in a sense of filial responsibility and willingness to support older relatives in need.
2. Three overlapping family dynamics contribute to filial responsibility during the emerging and young adult years: (a) role strain and unavailability on the part of the middle generation to take on elder caregiver roles, (b) expansion of the oldest cohort groups in families, and (c) intergenerational reciprocity—young adult family members wanting the opportunity to support elderly relatives who were active and involved in their lives as children.

These three family dynamics are described in greater detail next. Following that is a discussion of the findings from the only study, to our knowledge, that compares and contrasts emerging and young adult caregivers' and noncaregivers' attitudes toward filial responsibility.

FAMILY DYNAMICS CONTRIBUTING TO FILIAL RESPONSIBILITY

Middle Generation Role Strain

Recent national analyses confirm that the traditional caregivers to elderly relatives are mainly middle-aged women (Wolff & Kasper, 2006). These daughters and wives are described as under severe strain because they are "embedded with multiple and competing role demands and responsibilities" (Penning, 1998, p. S188). As outlined by Harris (1998), "In the last two decades as women have entered the workforce in unparalleled numbers, their commitment to caring for elderly members has not decreased" (p. 342). Wolff and Kasper (2006) estimated that as many as 50% of middle-aged caregivers face the challenge of juggling caregiving responsibilities with working and childrearing.

Our findings on emerging and young adult caregivers are consistent with the role strain previously attributed only to middle-aged caregivers. For more than half of the adult grandchildren participants in our research

(52%), their motivation to assume elder caregiver roles was directly linked to willingness to help their parents (Dellmann-Jenkins et al., 2000). A 21-year-old granddaughter stated, "I volunteered to care for my grandmother (age 81 years) in order help my mom." A 33-year-old granddaughter disclosed a more detailed and darker description of the dynamics of her acquisition of the elder care role to her 91-year-old grandmother:

> When Alzheimer's became apparent, my parents weren't coping well with it and were mean to her (not physically) . . . I couldn't stand it . . . I told them I would take her to my house. My dad told me it would be the biggest mistake I ever made. Three years later, I still disagree.

Our findings also revealed that 30% of the adult children reported that they received requests from other relatives (primarily middle-aged parents and siblings) to take on caregiver roles in order to keep the elderly relative living in the community (Dellmann-Jenkins & Brittain, 2003).

Expansion of the Oldest Generations in Families

The role strain experienced by many traditional elder caregivers is further compounded by the steadily increasing number of family members living into their 80s, 90s, and beyond. Recent demographic analyses (Poon, Jang, Reynolds, & McCarthy, 2005) have indicated that the age group 85 and older, often categorized as the "oldest old," is the fastest-growing segment of the U.S. population. This trend has resulted in an increase in the number of living generations, or what Harper (2005, p. 422) described as "intergenerational extension." Emerging and young adults are predicted to continue to take on primary caregiver roles to elderly relatives to help out the middle generations in their families (Giarrusso, Silverstein, & Bengtson, 1996; Levine et al., 2005). Young people with a strong sense of filial duty are a valuable resource in families where the middle generation often is already serving as a primary caregiver to an impaired older member and is unable to assume responsibility to yet an additional elderly relative (Dellmann-Jenkins et al., 2001).

Our findings on emerging and young adult caregivers are consistent with the family dynamic described above. A substantial number of the young adult caregivers in our research were grandchildren (49%) providing support to grandparents and great-grandparents in order to maintain the older generation's residence in the community (Dellmann-Jenkins et al., 2000). Furthermore, these granddaughters (44%) and grandsons (5%) were more likely to be living with their care recipient in order to avoid nursing home placement. However, it is important to note that the children (most of whom were young adults) and grandchildren (all of whom were emerging adults) participating in our research did not differ in their actual caregiving behaviors (Dellmann-Jenkins & Brittain, 2003; Dellmann-Jenkins et al., 2000). For example, the vast majority (90% to 100%) of children and grandchildren reported that they were providing assistance with transportation, companionship, and emotional support to the elderly care recipient on a daily basis. Four additional caregiving activities that were provided by most of the children and grandchildren included (a) making phone calls for the older relative regarding medical appointments, medication, and insurance reimbursements (60% to 65%); (b) household chores and preparing meals (85% to 95%); (c) attending to personal care needs of the older relative (55% to 65%); and (d) taking care of legal and financial matters (55% to 65%). These data are consistent with recent national analyses of emerging and young adults who are caregivers for elderly family members (Levine et al., 2005), middle-aged caregivers, and the types of support most frequently provided to elderly relatives.

Intergenerational Reciprocity

The link between willingness to take on an elder caregiver role and how involved the older generation was and is in the lives of the emerging and young adult generation has been documented. In a recent study, adult grandchildren were asked their motivations for taking on the elder caregiver role (Dellmann-Jenkins et al., 2001). "Wanting to return the love and nurturance received earlier by the grandparent" emerged as a central theme in their responses. A single 31-year-old providing daily care to her grandparents disclosed, "I am thankful I can do it. My mother was only 16 years old when I was born and my grandparents took care of me. I will never forget how she [my grandmother] *always* had time for me."

This young woman's sense of generational reciprocity would come as no surprise to Lillian Troll, a prominent researcher of three- and four-generational families. On the basis of her research, when families are under stress, grandparents move from their watchdog status to being active and involved in the lives of their grandchildren. According to Troll (1985), these grandparents, serving as caretakers, friends, and companions, can have an especially important and positive influence on the younger generation's emotional and psychological development. Although longitudinal research is needed that specifically tracks the impact of these early attachments with the older generation on emerging and young adults' later sense of filial duty, our cross-sectional findings suggest that when grandparents are under stress and at risk for nursing home placement, many emerging and young adults mirror the earlier behaviors of the older generation and move into active and involved elder caregiver roles (Dellmann-Jenkins et al., 2001).

The young caregivers' reports of positive outcomes resulting from their elder caregiving roles offer additional support for the family dynamic of intergenerational reciprocity. In our research, the most frequently reported benefit of the caregiving role by the adult grandchildren involved generational reciprocity and maintaining a close relationship with the older care recipient. One half of the grandchildren gave this response, and 18% of the young adult children reported this outcome. A college student revealed, "I enjoy talking to my grandfather about my family tree. He talks to me about my boyfriend and relationships." Another granddaughter said, "I get to talk to him about his life when he was younger. I am getting to know my family history. We get to go to games together." In addition to maintaining close ties, these young women and men viewed their caregiving role as an opportunity to reciprocate love and nurturance that had been received by them earlier in their relationship. Although the grandchildren (mostly emerging adults) most frequently reported that a benefit of their caregiver role was generational reciprocity and maintaining a close relationship with their older relative, the most frequently reported benefit of the young adult children was instrumental in nature. Over half of these participants (59%) acknowledged positive feelings as a result of avoiding nursing home placement for their older parents.

Caregivers' and Noncaregivers' Attitudes Toward Filial Responsibility

The purpose of the next section is to present further insight into emerging and young adults' views toward filial responsibility. This discussion is based on a study of young caregivers' and noncaregivers' attitudes toward filial responsibility (Dellmann-Jenkins & Brittain, 2003).

The sample consisted of 40 caregivers, from 18 to 40 years old, who were currently in caregiver roles to older relatives and 40 noncaregivers, also emerging and young adults, who had not yet assumed elder caregiver roles. The majority of the caregivers were young adults (26 to 40 years; 68%). The caregivers and noncaregivers did not differ in education, age, income, gender, race, or declared religious affiliation. One central theme emerged from the caregivers' responses when asked to describe the circumstances surrounding their decision to take on a primary caregiver role to an older relative: wanting to avoid nursing home placement. This objective was evident in all of their responses. The findings indicated that there were no differences between caregivers and noncaregivers in the belief that elderly relatives' negative traits should not affect one's sense of duty to support the older generation. Less consensus was found when comparing the two groups' responses to statements pertaining to home life and family relationships being disrupted as a result of caring for their older relatives. First, the caregivers were more likely than their noncaregiver peers to disagree with the statement, "Young adult family members should *not* care for elderly relatives if it makes for squabbling and turmoil in their homes all the time," $\chi^2(1, N = 30) = 32.9$, $p < .001$. Second, the caregivers were more likely than their noncaregiver peers to agree with the statement, "Adult children should provide a home for their elderly parents even if conflict arises between the older generation and grandchildren," $\chi^2(1, N = 30) = 28.5$, $p < .001$. Third, the caregivers were more likely than their noncaregiver peers to agree with the statement, "Older parents should be taken care of by their adult children regardless of the

feelings of their spouses," $\chi^2(1, N = 30) = 28.5, p < .001$. These group differences are intriguing and suggest that the young caregivers were willing
to tolerate the strained family relationships and stressful home environment that may result from accomplishing their key objective: avoiding
nursing home placement for their elderly relatives. What is not clear from
the data is the rationale for the caregivers' more tolerant responses.
Perhaps the caregivers were more tolerant of caregiving-related family
stress after having carefully analyzed the costs and rewards of assuming
the role. Or possibly, their responses of greater tolerance were the result
of cognitive mechanisms used to justify—if even just to themselves—why
they were in the stressful role.

The filial responsibility mean scores of the caregivers ($M = 67.7$) and
noncaregivers ($M = 65.9$) indicated that the two groups possessed similar
and positive attitudes toward helping older adults, as measured by
Ohuche and Littrell's (1989) survey of filial responsibility. In addition, the
majority of both groups (at least 50%) agreed with the three statements,
"We should look to the younger generation to support older family members," "Older family members should be able to look to younger relatives
for support when they are in need," and "Every child should be willing to
share their homes with their older parents." These findings demonstrate
greater consensus between the caregiver and noncaregiver groups in their
responses to these more general items than to the items more specific and
related to providing direct care discussed earlier. This suggests that vague
or general statements about family caregiving are more likely to be uni-
versally endorsed than are statements suggesting specific types of direct
family caregiving, the latter of which are supported more by young adults
who are actually in the caregiving role.

Young caregivers participating in this study had more positive
attitudes toward supporting older relatives than did their counterparts
in earlier studies (i.e., Dinkel, 1944; Ohuche & Littrel, 1989; Wake &
Sporakowski, 1972). In addition, the emerging and young adults' willingness to support older family members did not appear to be influenced by
their income or education. This finding supports Ohuche and Littrell
(1989), who concluded that a sense of duty to elderly relatives is intrinsic
and not directly affected by social class or level of formal education.

DELLMANN-JENKINS AND BLANKEMEYER

The intrinsic motivation may be rooted in a sense of filial responsibility—that is, a feeling of obligation to reciprocate care to their older relative—or it simply may be based on affection and desire to provide care to them (Stein et al., 1998).

The findings of this study do not substantiate the traditional view that a sense of obligation to help elderly relatives in need is unique to the middle years of adulthood. Emerging and young adult caregivers and noncaregivers possessed similar and positive attitudes toward helping older family members. Furthermore, the caregivers' main reason for taking on the role, to avoid nursing home placement for their elderly relative, helps to explain the significant differences between the two groups with respect to their responses to individual items in the filial responsibility scale. If future studies with larger and more representative samples of 18- to-40-year-olds generate similar data, earlier researchers' contentions that periods before middle adulthood are characterized by filial immaturity where a sense of duty or willingness to care for older family members has yet to develop (Blenkner, 1965) will need to be reworked.

EMERGING AND YOUNG ADULT FILIAL CAREGIVERS' RECOMMENDED SUPPORT SERVICES

The emerging and young adult caregivers in our research were asked which services would be most helpful to them in their caregiver role. Emotional support from others of the same age and in the same predicament was the most frequently needed service (as many as 50% of our participants made this request). The men and women who reported this need emphasized the value of home visits and visits over the phone as well as support groups, which focus primarily on giving moral support. One daughter who had revealed that she felt very isolated reported the need for "someone to come in and talk to me one-on-one or even over the phone. . . . I need to know that what I am going through is normal for the situation that I'm in; that I am not going crazy." The next most frequently needed service consisted of free or low-cost health care services to adults under 65 years. This was reported by about 40% of the participants. A daughter caring for her father painfully disclosed, "It is such a strain to see him not have enough funds for his medication. It's heart-breaking to see him make choices between survival needs like food and housing, or his health." Third, at least 40% of the young caregivers participating in our research wished that they were involved in a support group. On the basis of our qualitative data, support group meetings are likely to be most beneficial when they provide moral support and guidance on how to cope with six key caregiving stressors: (a) lack of time to establish or maintain intimate relationships, (b) added strain in the early stages of marriage, (c) balancing the care of very young children with elder care roles, (d) meeting the demands of early career development or coping with having to postpone one's career aspirations, (e) premature role reversal with one's parents, and (f) failure to establish emotional independence from the family of origin. The range of role strain young adult caregivers may be experiencing was described by a 26-year-old man caring for his father: "I have recently married, I am trying to deal with a new family, my sister is impossible, and I just moved to a new city. Boy, am I stressed!" As a result of the caregivers' responses, we suggest that support groups be designed to specifically meet the oftentimes "demographically dense" lives of emerging and young adult caregivers. Levine et al. (2005) identified several support groups specifically designed for emerging to young adult caregivers, including Alzheimer's Association chapters in the states of New Jersey and New York, and concluded that these may provide models for others.

A substantial number (33%) of the emerging and young adults in our research reported increased church attendance and participation in religious groups as a result of their caregiver roles. These findings substantiate Levine et al.'s (2005) recommendation that religious organizations provide targeted outreach, information, and special programs for emerging and young adult caregivers. These researchers also recommended that clergy leaders collaborate and create joint programs if there are not enough young caregivers in a single congregation to form a program.

Human resource personnel are also encouraged to offer targeted support and information to emerging and young adult employees who are in elder caregiving roles. Many of the emerging and young adults (at least 40%) participating in our research reported problems with workplace attendance and job performance as outcomes of their caregiving roles. Access to counselors and elder care case managers located at the work site may help alleviate emotional strains and provide instrumental support, such as information on free or low-cost health care services for the older care recipients and support groups for emerging and young adult caregivers. In addition, human resource personnel who advocate for these young elder caregivers could enlist the assistance of management to implement flexible work schedules and flexible leave time. Options such as work sharing, leave sharing, and personal leave time could substantially reduce the negative impact experienced by emerging and young adult caregivers in the area of career development.

RECOMMENDATIONS FOR FUTURE RESEARCH AND CONCLUSIONS

Research involving larger and more demographically diverse samples of emerging and young adult caregivers than provided in our research is needed to draw more conclusive results about the early acquisition of the elder caregiver role. Data from two national surveys of young caregivers indicate representative proportions of caregivers by race (e.g., 15% of young caregivers were Hispanic and 14% to 16% were African American; Levine et al., 2005). Race and ethnicity should be considered when assessing the effects of the caregiving role on progression through developmental tasks because timing of developmental tasks varies by race (e.g., U.S. Census Bureau, 2001) as do values related to development itself (e.g., individualism versus collectivism; Gilovich, Wang, Regan, & Sadafumi, 2003). Racially and ethnically diverse populations of young caregivers also should be included in future studies because research on traditional aged caregivers shows differences by race in rates of assuming the caregiving role (e.g., American Association of Retired Persons, 2004) and in caregiving experiences. For example, the findings of the Navaie-Waliser et al. (2001) study suggest that Black caregivers are apt to more provide more intense care than White caregivers and also experience heightened religious practice after assuming their caregiving roles. Racial and ethnic factors also should be considered when examining the rationale behind young adults' decision to assume the caregiving role. Levine et al. (2005) concluded that national studies specifically designed to gather data on emerging and young adult caregivers are needed.

In addition, studies securing comparison groups of emerging and young adult filial caregivers with noncaregivers would provide a clearer picture of how well the caregivers accomplish important developmental tasks compared with other emerging and young adults who are not providing care to an older impaired relative. Furthermore, comparisons across emerging adults, young adults, and traditional-age caregivers (adults in their mid-40s to mid-60s) would shed light on the direct effect of the caregivers' age, and the issue of whether emerging and young adult caregivers experience more difficulties than older caregivers could also be addressed. Similarly, the effect of caregivers' age on the reported positive outcomes could be identified. Also, the effect of age on caregiving motivations and attitudes toward filial obligation could be determined. Some research shows that young people report higher levels of willingness to care for aged relatives than their middle-aged counterparts (Wake & Sporakowski, 1972).

Finally, longitudinal research is needed on the development of individuals who acquire the elder caregiver role very early in adulthood in terms of other family roles (e.g., marital, parental) and personal decisions (e.g., career, further education). Such studies may provide valuable information on (a) the long-term development of adults who assume elder care responsibilities earlier than normal, (b) possible missed opportunities in terms of career and the development of intimate relationships, as well as (c) positive family relationship outcomes and personal rewards. Longitudinal research should also address the issue of what happens to these young caregivers when the elder care ceases. Levine et al. (2005) noted that longitudinal studies are necessary to examine how family caregiving affects emerging young adults and how the impact differs on the basis of gender, race and ethnicity, and relationship to the older care recipient.

In conclusion, one of the major strengths of our research (Dellmann-Jenkins et al., 2000, 2001; Dellmann-Jenkins & Brittain, 2003) is that it draws attention to the increasing population of emerging and young adults providing assistance to older family members and the potential impact of acquiring the elder caregiving role on developmental tasks typical of 18- to 40-year-olds. An additional strength of this research program is our data, which suggest that providing assistance to elderly family members offers an opportunity for young caregivers to experience positive family and personal outcomes, such as increased closeness with the care recipient and enhanced feelings of self-respect and competency, as well as the more commonly acknowledged negative outcomes. Our research also substantiates the use of both qualitative and quantitative data collection methods. Inclusion of both methodologies has allowed us to better understand emerging and young adults' filial responsibility toward elderly relatives and the potential impact of their caregiving roles on intimacy and career decisions, marriage, and family life demands.

REFERENCES

American Association of Retired Persons. (2004). *A report of multicultural boomers coping with family and aging issues.* Washington, DC: Author.

Arnett, J. J. (2000). Emerging adulthood: A theory of development from the late teens through the twenties. *American Psychologist, 55,* 469–480.

Arnett, J. J. (2001). Conceptions of the transition to adulthood: Perspectives from adolescence through midlife. *Journal of Adult Development, 8,* 133–143.

Arnett, J. J. (2004). *Emerging adulthood.* New York: Oxford University Press.

Arnett, J. J., & Tanner, J. L. (2006). *Emerging adults in America: Coming of age in the 21st century.* Washington, DC: American Psychological Association.

Azar, S. T. (2003). Adult development and parenthood: A social–cognitive perspective. In J. Demick & C. Andreoletti (Eds.), *Handbook of adult development* (pp. 391–415). New York: Kluwer.

Baltes, P. B. (1987). Theoretical propositions of life-span developmental psychology: On the dynamics of growth and decline. *Developmental Psychology, 23,* 611–626.

Baltes, P. B., Lindenberger, U., & Staudinger, U. M. (1998). Life-span theory in developmental psychology. In R. M. Lerner (Ed.), *Handbook of child psychology: Vol. 1. Theoretical models of human development* (pp. 1029–1143). New York: Wiley.

Barnett, R. C., & Marshall, N. L. (1992a). Men's job and partner roles: Spillover effects and psychological distress. *Sex Roles, 27,* 455–472.

Barnett, R. C., & Marshall, N. L. (1992b). Worker and mother roles, spillover effects and psychological distress. *Women and Health, 18,* 9–40.

Barton, P. E. (2002). *The closing of the education frontier?* Princeton, NJ: Educational Testing Service.

Blenkner, M. (1965). Social work and family relationships in later life with some thoughts on filial maturity. In E. Shanas & G. F. Streib (Eds.), *Social structure and the family* (pp. 46–59), Englewood Cliffs, NJ: Prentice-Hall.

Camp, P., & Ganong, L. (1997). Locus of control and marital satisfaction in long-term marriages. *Families in Society, 77,* 624–631.

Carstensen, L. L. (1992). Social and emotional patterns in adulthood: Support for socioemotional selectivity theory. *Psychology and Aging, 7,* 331–338.

Crittenden, A. (2001). *The price of motherhood: Why the most important job in the world is still undervalued.* New York: Metropolitan.

Dellmann-Jenkins, M., Blankemeyer, M., & Pinkard, O. (2000). Young adult children and grandchildren in primary caregiver roles to older relatives and their service needs. *Family Relations, 49,* 177–186.

Dellmann-Jenkins, M., Blankemeyer, M., & Pinkard, O. (2001). Incorporating the elder caregiving role into the developmental tasks of young adulthood. *International Journal of Aging and Human Development, 52,* 1–18.

Dellmann-Jenkins, M., & Brittain, L. (2003). Young adults' attitudes toward filial responsibility and actual assistance to elderly family members. *Journal of Applied Gerontology, 22*(2), 21–229.

Dinkel, R. (1944). Attitudes of children toward supporting aged parents. *American Sociological Review, 9,* 370–379.

Erikson, E. H. (1968). *Identity: Youth and crisis.* New York: Norton.

Erikson, E. H. (1980). *Identity and the life cycle.* New York: Norton.

Erikson, E. H. (1982). *The life cycle completed.* New York: Norton.

Fuligni, A., & Pedersen, S. (2002). Family obligation and the transition to young adulthood. *Developmental Psychology, 38,* 856–868.

Giarrusso, R., Silverstein, M., & Bengtson, V. (1996). Family complexity and the grandparent role. *Generations,* 17–23.

Gilovich, T., Wang, R. F., Regan, D., & Sadafumi, N. (2003). Regrets of action and inaction across cultures. *Journal of Cross-Cultural Psychology, 34,* 61–71.

Goldscheider, F., & Goldscheider, C. (1999). *The changing transition to adulthood: Leaving and returning home.* Thousand Oaks, CA: Sage.

Harper, S. (2005). Grandparenthood. In M. L. Johnson (Ed.), *The Cambridge handbook of age and ageing* (pp. 422–428).New York: Cambridge University Press.

Harris, P. (1998) Listening to caregiving sons. *The Gerontologist, 38,* 342–352.

Levine, C., Hunt, G. G., Halper, D., Hart, A. Y., Lautz, J., & Gould, D. A. (2005). Young adult caregivers: A first look at an unstudied population. *American Journal of Public Health, 95,* 2071–2075.

Lino, M. (2002). *Expenditures on children by families, 2001. Annual Report.* (Miscellaneous Publication No. 1528—2001.) Washington DC: U.S. Department of Agriculture, Center for Nutrition Policy and Promotion.

Martin, J. A., Hamilton, B. E., Sutton, P. D., Ventura, S., Menacker, F., & Munson, M. (2003, December 17). Births: Final data for 2002. *National Vital Statistics Report, 52*(10), Hyattsville, MD: National Center for Health Statistics.

Moen, P. (1999). *The Cornell Couples and Careers Study.* Ithaca, NY: Cornell University.

Navaie-Waliser, M., Feldman, P., Gould, D., Levine, C., Kuerbis, A., & Donelan, K. (2001). The experiences and challenges of informal caregivers: Common themes and differences among Whites, Blacks, and Hispanics. *The Gerontologist, 41,* 733–214.

Ohuche, N., & Littrell, J. (1989). Igbo students' attitudes toward supporting aged parents. *International Journal of Aging and Human Development, 29,* 259–267.

Papalia, D. E., Olds, S. W., & Feldman, R. D. (2007). *Human development* (10th ed.). New York: McGraw-Hill.

Penning, M. (1998). In the middle: Parent caregiving in the context of other roles. *Journal of Gerontology, 53B*(4), S188–S197.

Poon, L. W., Jang, Y., Reynolds, S., & McCarthy, E. (2005). Profiles of the oldest-old. In M. L. Johnson (Ed.), *The Cambridge handbook of age and ageing* (pp. 346–353). New York: Cambridge University Press.

Santrock, J. W. (2007). *A topical approach to life-span development.* New York: McGraw-Hill.

Sax, L. J. Lindholm, J. A., Astin, A. W., Korn, W. S., & Mahoney, K. M. (2002). *The American freshman: National norms for fall 2002.* Los Angeles: University of California, Higher Education Research Institute.

Schaie, K. W., & Willis, S. L. (2002). *Adult development and aging.* Upper Saddle River, NJ: Prentice Hall.

Scharf, M., Mayseless, O., & Kivenson-Baron, I. (2004). Adolescents' attachment representations and developmental tasks in emerging adulthood. *Developmental Psychology, 40,* 430–444.

Schulenberg, J. E., Bryant, A. L., & O'Malley, P. M. (2004). Taking hold of some kind of life: How developmental tasks relate to trajectories of well-being during the transition to adulthood. *Development and Psychopathology, 16,* 1119–1140.

Shifren, K. (2001). Early caregiving and adult depression: Good news for young caregivers. *The Gerontologist, 41,* 188–190.

Shifren, K., & Kachorek, L. V. (2003). Does early caregiving matter? The effects on young caregivers' adult mental health. *International Journal of Behavioral Development, 27,* 338–346.

Stein, C. H., Wemmerus, V. A., Ward, M., Gaines, M. E., Freeberg, A. L., & Jewell, T. C. (1998). "Because they're my parents": An intergenerational study of felt obligation and parental caregiving. *Journal of Marriage and Family, 60,* 611–22.

Teachman J. D., & Paasch, K. (1998). The family and educational aspirations. *Journal of Marriage and the Family, 60,* 704–714.

Troll, L. (1985). The contingencies of grandparenting. In V. L. Bengtson & J. F. Robertson (Eds.), *Grandparenthood* (pp. 135–149). Thousand Oaks, CA: Sage.

Twenge, J. M., Campbell, W. K., & Foster, C. (2003). Parenthood and marital satisfaction: A meta-analytic review. *Journal of Marriage and the Family, 65,* 574–583.

U.S. Census Bureau. (2001). *Survey of income and program participation (SIPP), 2001 panel, Wave 2 topical module.* Retrieved July 22, 2006, from http://www.census.gov/population/socdemo/hh-fam/ms2.xls

U.S. Census Bureau. (2005). *Current population survery.* Retrieved July 22, 2006, from http://www.census.gov/population/socdemo/education/cps2004/tab01a-01.pdf

U.S. Census Bureau. (2006). *Table MS-2. Estimated median age at first marriage, by sex: 1890 to the present.* Retrieved April 18, 2008, from http://www.census.gov/population/socdemo/hh-fam/ms2.xls

Verbrugge, L. M. (1989). The twain meet: Empirical explanations of sex differences in health and mortality. *Journal of Health and Social Behavior, 30,* 282–304.

Wake, S., & Sporakowski, M. (1972). An intergenerational comparison of attitudes towards supporting aged parents. *Journal of Marriage and the Family, 34,* 42–48.

Ward, R., & Spitze, G. (2007). Nestleaving and coresidence of young adult children. *Research on Aging, 29, 257–277.*

White, L. (1994). Coresidence and leaving home: Young adults and their parents. *Annual Review of Sociology, 20,* 81–102.

Wolff, J. L. & Kasper, J. D. (2006). Caregivers of frail elders: Updating a national profile. *The Gerontologist, 46,* 344–356.

Wolfsen, C., Hanfield-Jones, R., Glass, K., McClaren, J., & Keyserlingk, E. (1993). Adult children's perceptions of their responsibility to provide care for dependent elderly parents. *The Gerontologist, 33,* 315–323.

4

"I Owe It To Them": Understanding Felt Obligation Toward Parents in Adulthood

Catherine H. Stein

My mother would sometimes joke that she was happy that she had a daughter because there would always be someone around to take care of her in her old age—in the style to which she had become accustomed. But I knew that she wasn't really kidding.

—Arlene, age 51, daughter, wife, and mother

For the first time in history, relationships between children and their parents are primarily situated in adulthood, with adults typically spending more than 50 years relating to their parents (Hagestad, 1991). In the United States, an individual is now likely to spend more years being an adult child with living parents than being a parent of a minor child (Watkins, Menken, & Bongaarts, 1987). Implications of an aging society are not gender neutral because women typically assume primary roles in "kinkeeping" and caring for elder family members (Walker, 1992).

Scholars have increasingly recognized the importance of studying family relationships across the adult life course. Yet our understanding of the obligations that surround adults' relations with their parents is surprisingly limited. Research has focused primarily on general attitudes toward adults' responsibility to care for their infirm parents, without consideration for the

I thank the women and men who participated in research studies of felt obligation and the doctoral students in the clinical psychology program at Bowling Green State University who assisted me in conducting these studies. I extend my appreciation to my husband, Mark Baron, for his support and helpful feedback on an initial version of the chapter and to my son, Matthew Carlos Baron, for his patience, thoughtfulness, and sense of humor.

development and enactment of obligations that unfold across time within the context of adults' ongoing relationships with their parents.

In the present chapter, I examine theory and research on adults' obligation toward their parents and explore the role of obligation in parental caregiving across the life course. Rather than conceptualizing parental obligation as a general attitude, I have studied felt obligation as a set of rights and duties that occur within the context of adults' ongoing relationships with parents across the life course. The major assumptions of a life course perspective and feminist views of caregiving are reviewed in this chapter to place the study of felt obligation in a larger theoretical context. Research is presented that illustrates the usefulness of felt obligation in describing adults' reports of parental caregiving. Studies of young, middle-aged, and older adults that examine differences in felt obligation as a function of gender and phase of life are reviewed. The implications of research findings on felt obligation for the study of child–parent relationships in adulthood and for future research directions are discussed.

FAMILY OBLIGATION: TAKING A LIFE COURSE PERSPECTIVE

A life course perspective acknowledges the personal, social, and historical contexts that shape the lives of individuals. Life course scholars attempt to describe social structures and pathways that organize human experience and identify aspects of continuity and change in adult lives over time. A life course perspective begins with a set of fundamental propositions about the nature of human development and the factors that most influence it (for an excellent overview of life course principles, see Settersten, 2003). Personal and historical time, chronological age, and social interconnectedness are life course concepts that have important implications for the study of family obligation.

The concept of time is essential to a life course perspective of human development (Alwin, 1995). The life course can be viewed as age-linked periods such as childhood, youth, young adulthood, middle adulthood, and old age (Hagestad & Neugarten, 1985). It is assumed that individual development does not stop at young adulthood but continues throughout life.

Some developmental processes are thought to be continuous and extend across the life course, and others are thought to be unique to certain periods and discontinuous over time. Social and cultural expectations about developmental tasks, social roles, activities, and experiences are associated with certain periods in life. For example, the developmental tasks of young adulthood in the United States typically include living independently from parents, getting a job or pursuing postsecondary education, getting married, and having children. These types of social constructions about the life course are said to be used by individuals as social timetables to organize their own lives and the lives of others (Settersten & Hagestad, 1996). Both individuals and family members may experience substantial distress as a result of deviating from social expectations, such as deciding to marry later in life, being married and deciding not to have children, or choosing to become a single parent. Dominant cultural expectations about the life course can provide a sense of order and predictability in the lives of individuals (Hagestad, 1996) but can also serve as mechanisms for social control and oppression of social groups (Baber & Allen, 1992; Rappaport, 1995).

Life course scholars contend that specific periods of life must be understood in the context of individuals' lived experience and anticipated future (Settersten, 2003). In other words, histories, circumstances, plans, and dreams constantly impact people's lives. As importantly, people have other people, and the histories, circumstances, and dreams of significant others also connect us and shape our experience. Life course scholars use the term *linked lives* to convey the notion that people's lives are intimately connected and influenced by the lives of others (Greenfield & Marks, 2006). Of course, both the paths of individuals and the collective lives of cohorts of people are marked by the larger circumstances of culture and history (Hareven, 1991).

Framing the study of family obligation in life course terms means paying considerable attention to how concepts such as interdependence, age, life phase, and history shape relationships among family members across time. These notions are central to the study of families because relationships with kin are assumed to be lifelong and exist, by definition, within a unique context of previous history and future involvement. Family relationships are negotiated against the backdrop of social and cultural expectations about the "normal" family at each period of the life course (Rindfuss, Swicegood, & Rosenfeld, 1987; Stein & Wemmerus, 2001).

ATTITUDINAL AND RELATIONAL APPROACHES TO THE STUDY OF FAMILY OBLIGATION

Family obligation has not exactly been a hot topic in social science research. In part, this lack of research interest reflects a historical shift in the characterization of the American family by the late 19th century. In a primarily agricultural America, the family was an economic unit wherein parents and children took responsibility for farming and received income from production (Schorr, 1980). Kinship roles were relatively structured, and family survival was largely dependent on mutual obligations among family members. American expansion and the industrial revolution brought new economic opportunities that allowed children greater autonomy from parents and emphasized emancipation from family. Family went from being viewed as set of relations governed by rights and duties to a set of social ties based on personal choice and affection (Hareven, 1986). In this contemporary view, adults maintain relationships with family because they "want to" and not because they "have to." Kin relations are seen as being motivated by affection and intimacy, and family associations are thought to reflect a high degree of personal discretion.

Those researchers interested in family obligation typically conceptualize it as a general attitude or societal norm regarding family ties. When asked about the duties that "people in general" hold toward relatives, adults have consistently endorsed contact and assistance as strong social expectations of kinship (Adams, 1968; Reiss, 1962). Adults typically have reported higher levels of general obligation for the roles of parents and children than for other family roles, such as that of siblings or in-laws, and have reported strong negative sanctions for nonperformance of kinship obligations (Adams, 1968; Bahr, 1976).

In the early 1980s, research on family obligation began to focus on adults' duties as caregivers to elderly parents. The concept of filial responsibility became the dominant view of family obligation among researchers. *Filial responsibility* is defined as an attitude about a set of responsibilities or obligations that adult children should assume when parents are old and infirm (Hanson, Sauer, & Seelbach, 1983; Seelbach, 1984). Studies have shown that both parents and adult children have expectations regarding filial responsibility (Gelfand, 1989; Hamon & Blieszner, 1990) and that filial responsibility differs as a function of geographic distance from parents, race, and residential location (rural vs. urban; Finley, Roberts, & Banahan, 1988; Hanson et al., 1983).

As an attitudinal approach to the study of obligation, filial responsibility emphasizes the larger social context in which duties between adults and their parents may unfold. However, the concept of filial responsibility limits the study of obligation in a number of important ways. Filial responsibility assumes that family obligation is salient in one period of the life course, when parents reach old age. Filial responsibility is triggered by parental infirmity and need. Pervasive social attitudes about duty toward aged parents will motivate adults' behavior toward parents when parental need inevitably arises. This perpetuates the idea that aging is synonymous with decline and that accompanying burdens are to be endured by family. The personal histories of children and their parents and the lifelong nature of child–parent relationships are almost entirely ignored by this approach to obligation. In fact, filial responsibility says nothing about the specific expectations for behavior that adults develop in their ongoing relationships with their parents over the life course.

In contrast, relational approaches to the study of obligation see family relationships as central to understanding kin duties and responsibilities. A relational approach recognizes the existence of social norms but emphasizes that adults must apply norms about obligation in the context of their ongoing family relationships (Finch, 1989; Stein, 1992). Obligation toward kin is often viewed as "negotiated commitments," which emerge between family members in adulthood as they decide what things they do and do not do in their relationships. These negotiations can be implicit or explicit and are not necessarily conducted at the level of conscious strategy (Finch, 1989; Stein 1992).

Using a relational approach, my colleagues and I define *felt obligation* as expectations for appropriate behavior as perceived within the context of specific personal relationships with kin across the life course (Stein, 1992;

Stein et al., 1998). Felt obligation is not limited to a single expectation but is multidimensional in nature. In our work, we find that felt obligation is negotiated across a number of relevant relationship domains. Felt obligation is not viewed as an exclusively negative aspect of relationships but rather is seen as a set of practical "oughts" and "shoulds" that guide adults' interactions with parents. Dimensions of felt obligation reflect the fundamental importance of both separation and connectedness issues between children and parents in adulthood (Stein, 1993).

The duties to provide needed assistance and maintain contact are fundamental to most operational definitions of family obligation (Hanson et al., 1983; Seelbach & Sauer, 1977) and are included as two dimensions of felt obligation. Given the negative sanctions against severing family ties, the need to avoid conflict in interactions with parents may also be quite strong. Moreover, expectations about appropriate levels of communication and personal sharing become salient when a lifetime of personal involvement is assumed. For example, older parents expect their adult children to maintain open and honest lines of communication with them, and expectations about sharing important matters are reported by both older parents and their adult children (Blieszner & Mancini, 1987; Hamon & Blieszner, 1990). Adults and parents are likely to negotiate expectations about the kinds of personal information that they should share and should avoid in interactions with one another. The responsibilities of adults to avoid conflict and share information about important matters with parents are included as two additional aspects of felt obligation.

Adult relationships with parents are likely to involve issues surrounding individuation as well as connectedness. Social norms regarding independence of children in adulthood enhance expectations about self-sufficiency and place limits on personal sharing and communication in interactions with parents. The obligation to maintain appropriate levels of self-sufficiency is also included as a dimension of felt obligation. In summary, we conceptualize felt obligation as consisting of five dimensions that include a duty to maintain appropriate levels of contact, assistance, avoidance of interpersonal conflict, personal sharing, and self-sufficiency.

Relational and attitudinal approaches make opposite predictions about the importance of obligation toward parents for individuals at different points in their adult lives. By definition, filial responsibility assumes that kin duties are salient to adults when parents are elderly, infirm, and in need of assistance. Obligation emerges from the societal expectations that elderly parents have a "right" to be taken care of and that adult children have a "duty" toward their parents to do so when parents are in need. Thus, parental obligation becomes an issue for adult children in middle age and later life when aging parents have need for care.

Relational approaches, in contrast, assume that obligation toward parents is related to sacrifices that parents make in childrearing that are acknowledged in adulthood. The nonreciprocal flow of resources from parent to child during childhood is thought to be associated with a personal sense of indebtedness to parents in adulthood. Duties performed by adult children over the life course serve as "repayment" for parental sacrifices, which helps to alleviate a sense of personal indebtedness and to increase feelings of reciprocity over time (Rossi & Rossi, 1990; Stein, 1993). Felt obligation is assumed to have important implications for individuals' relationships with parents early in the adult life course. From this perspective, young adults would be expected to express higher levels of felt obligation than middle-aged adults because young adults would have relatively fewer opportunities to "repay" parents than would their middle-aged counterparts.

Previous qualitative research on kin obligation (Stein & Rappaport, 1986) and theoretical discussions of obligation from sociology and psychology (Adams, 1968; Bahr, 1976; Karpel & Strauss, 1983) led to the development of the Felt Obligation Measure (FOM; Stein, 1992), a 34-item self-report instrument designed to tap adults' expectations regarding appropriate interactions in relationships with kin. Items for the measure were generated to reflect issues of separation and connectedness in adult relations.

Using a 5-point Likert scale, the FOM asks respondents to rate how often they feel they "need to" or "should" do or say particular things in their relationships with specific family members such as parents. Felt obligation is operationalized as the frequency with which adults report particular expectations (defined as a "need" or a "should") in their ongoing relationship with a specified (target) family member. In addition to an overall score of felt obligation, the FOM yields scores on five empirically derived subscales that assess expectations regarding contact and family ritual, assistance, conflict avoidance, personal sharing, and self-sufficiency. Reliability and construct validity data suggest that the FOM has good psychometric properties (for further description of the instrument, see Stein, 1992). The research on felt obligation that I describe in this chapter used the FOM to assess felt obligation toward parents at various periods in the adult life course.

DUTIFUL DAUGHTERS: PARENTAL CAREGIVING, HELPING, AND FELT OBLIGATION

The predominance of women as caregivers is among the most consistent findings in social science research on the family. Women typically assume the role of kinkeepers, being centrally involved in maintaining family contact and cohesion within and across generations (Coward & Dwyer, 1990; Hooyman & Gonyea, 1995). Women provide more hours of care to frail elders than do men and provide older relatives with a greater variety of assistance (Walker, 1992). Daughters are more likely than sons to provide routine care for elderly parents, with daughters typically outnumbering sons by more than 3 to 1 (Horowitz, 1985). In general, sons are more likely to assist parents with activities of daily living if daughters, daughters-in-law, or more distant female relatives are unavailable (Hooyman & Gonyea, 1995). Research suggests that sons provide more intermittent care than daughters and are more likely to withdraw from care as parents become increasingly disabled (Matthews & Rosner, 1988; Stoller, 1990).

Caregiving research typically assesses the degree to which parents rely on their adult children for assistance with routine daily activities such as bathing, dressing, and grooming when parents are infirm or disabled. Studies have also assessed the degree to which adult children provide help with instrumental activities of daily living to parents such as shopping, cooking, housework, transportation, and making doctors' appointments. Researchers have sometimes included the assessment of emotional supports in defining caregiving such as advice giving, listening, and problem solving. Authors have argued that activities defined as *parental caregiving* can simply be considered as a subset of helping exchanges between adults and their parents (Laditka & Laditka, 2001; Spitze & Logan, 1992). Calling these activities *helping exchanges* rather than *caregiving* avoids any pejorative connotation associated with the term *caregiving* and allows researchers to better study exchanges between adult children and parents across the life course. It has also been argued that restricting the study of adult–parent exchanges to assisting infirm or disabled parents with activities of daily living may underrepresent sons' helping roles and limit an understanding of the range of help provided by daughters (Laditka & Laditka, 2001; Stoller, 1990).

Sons tend to fare slightly better in studies of parental helping than they do in studies of parental caregiving. Sons are generally more likely than daughters to repair or make things for both mothers and fathers (Rossi & Rossi, 1990). Helping tasks performed by sons for older parents typically include yard work, household repairs, and management of finances (Hochschild, 1989; Stoller, 1990). Spitze and Logan (1992) found no significant gender differences in adults' reports of providing instrumental support to parents who were under the age of 75. This study found that mothers generally received more help from children than fathers, but mother–son pairs were not significantly different from mother–daughter pairs in the likelihood of a child helping a parent. When Spitze and Logan (1990) directly compared the role of gender in parental helping and support, they found that the key to parents receiving help from adult children is having at least one daughter, with no advantage of additional children of either gender. The research found little evidence of sons "substituting" for daughters in intergenerational helping. The authors concluded that sons do not easily assume helping tasks under most circumstances where daughters are unavailable.

Feminist scholars articulate family caregiving as a women's issue. Although there are different forms of feminist theory, a feminist perspective emphasizes the primarily socially constructed and not biologically determined nature of family care. Feminist scholars assert that a failure to challenge deeply held societal beliefs about women's "natural" role as family caregivers perpetuates gender stratification and the oppression of women in both public and private sectors of society (Hooyman & Gonyea, 1995).

Gender as a social construct is a form of classification based on social values that structure the opportunities and constraints experienced by individuals across the life course (Stoller, 1994). More than the biological category of sex, gender is a label given to individuals and an aspect of a hierarchical social structure that forges individual identities and shapes the personal aspirations, goals, and activities of everyday life (Stoller, 1994).

Feminist scholars have criticized social science researchers for using gender-neutral terms such as *caregiver, parent,* and *spouse* in studies of family caring, rather than terms such as *woman, mother,* and *wife* (Abel & Nelson, 1990; Traustadottir, 1991). When researchers analyze and report gender differences, these differences are typically conceptualized as properties of individuals rather than principles of social structure or institutional oppression. Abel (1989) described caregiving as both a profound personal experience and an oppressive social institution. As McGraw and Walker (2004) noted, a feminist perspective sensitizes researchers to the importance of women's experiences in both providing and receiving care. Caregiving can be experienced simultaneously as a burden and a gift, with the unpaid labor of caregiving consuming time and depleting resources while promoting individual satisfaction, personal control, power, and connectedness within the family (Di Leonardo, 1987; Graham, 1985). Much has been written about the burdens associated with caregiving (Hooyman & Gonyea, 1995), but a systematic understanding of the benefits associated with providing care or the aspects of family relationships that motivate caregiving across the adult life course is limited.

My colleagues and I have found consistent differences in men's and women's reports of felt obligation toward their parents across the life course. Women generally have reported higher overall levels of felt obligation and have scored significantly higher on most dimensions of felt obligation than have men (Stein, 1992; Stein et al., 1998). We have found that gender differences in reports of felt obligation toward parents generally hold for young and middle-aged adult samples (Stein et al., 1998). Both men and women generally have reported more felt obligation toward mothers than toward fathers (Stein, 1992; Stein & Ward, 1997). For example, both men and women in young adulthood generally reported higher levels of obligation toward their mothers than their fathers on the dimensions of contact and family ritual, assistance, conflict avoidance, and self-sufficiency (Stein, 1992). On only one dimension of felt obligation, personal sharing, did young adult women differ from men. Daughters were significantly more likely than sons to report that they felt obligated to engage in personal sharing with their mothers.

Giving voice to the experiences of women is paramount in a feminist research agenda. Much of what is known about family caregiving comes exclusively from the perspective of women. Women are overwhelmingly the participants in research surveys and interviews about family caregiving (Hooyman & Gonyea, 1995). A danger in this imbalance in research participation is that the roles that men play in the process of family care are either invisible or constantly defined relative to the caregiving roles and activities of women. However, socially constructed definitions of women as "natural caregivers" affect both men's and women's lives.

In studying felt obligation toward parents in adulthood, my colleagues and I include the views of both men and women whenever possible. Limiting the focus of research to women makes it difficult to disentangle the role of gender in felt obligation and the implications of parental obligation in family life. For example, in a study of young married couples, wives generally reported higher overall levels of obligation toward their mother and their father than did husbands (Stein, 1992). However, felt obligation toward parents was associated with significantly higher levels of self-reported depression, neuroticism, and global severity of psychological symptoms for husbands, but not for wives. Why would felt obligation toward parents in young adulthood be related to psychological distress for men but not for women? Such results may speak to the gendered nature of caregiving. There may be more opportunities for daughters to discharge feelings of obligation by enacting family responsibilities than there are for sons. Enactment of felt obligation may serve to help repay parents for sacrifices made in childrearing, thereby alleviating a woman's sense of personal indebtedness and increasing feelings of reciprocity in a woman's relationship with parents over time. Such findings are intriguing and highlight the complex nature of adult child–parent ties for both sons and daughters. More research is needed to understand the differential benefits of caregiving for women and men.

When it comes to predicting caregiving, investigators have identified parental affection as well as parental obligation as a possible motive for adult children (Cicirelli, 1993; Quinn, 1983). The notion here is that emotional closeness and affection are what primarily drive adults to provide care. The nature of the relationship between filial obligation and parental affection has been the subject of debate. Authors have varyingly asserted that filial obligation emerges from affection in family relations (Jarrett, 1985), that filial obligation and affection reflect different motivations for providing care (Finley et al., 1988), and that filial obligation and affection occur simultaneously as adult children contemplate parental caregiving (Walker, Pratt, Shinn, & Jones, 1990).

Unfortunately, little is known about gender differences in obligation and affection as motives for parental caregiving. Empirical studies have typically focused on relationships between filial responsibility, affection, and caregiving of elderly women by their adult daughters. In his summary of research findings, Cicirelli (1993) suggested that for women already providing care, higher levels of parental affection were associated with lower levels of filial responsibility. In contrast, affection and filial responsibility appeared to be positively related in studies in which daughters were not presently engaged in caregiving.

In terms of theory, a feminist perspective challenges researchers to consider the personal and societal implications of gender and family care. However, the questions that researchers ask and the research designs that they use need to be able to address the differential effects of gender on family life. Methodologically, gender can be considered as a fundamental base-rate variable against which the usefulness of other family variables related to parental caregiving can be evaluated. In other words, for a family variable to be useful in describing parental caregiving, it should be able to account for more variance in reports of parental caregiving than would simply knowing the gender of respondents.

FELT OBLIGATION, AFFECTION, FILIAL RESPONSIBILITY: GENDER AND LIFE COURSE ISSUES

My colleagues and I have conducted several studies to describe aspects of felt obligation at different periods of the life course and to establish the psychometric properties of the FOM. An intergenerational study conducted with 460 young adults and their middle-aged parents (Stein et al., 1998) merits review because it highlights gender and life course issues related to felt obligation and parental caregiving. We examined differences and similarities in adults' reports of felt obligation as a function of gender, generation (young, middle age), and parent status (one or two living parents). We also investigated whether adults' reports of felt obligation could account for variation in their reports of parental caregiving beyond the variance attributable to the gender of the adult child. The study was also the first to directly compare the role of felt obligation, filial responsibility, and parental affection in accounting for variation in adults' reports of parental caregiving. Our overarching goal was to examine the usefulness of felt obligation relative to other established family constructs in describing intergenerational relationships between adults and their parents.

Young adults and their middle-aged parents who participated in the study were separately asked to complete self-report measures of felt obligation, filial responsibility, parental affection, and caregiving in their relationships with their parents (for study details, see Stein et al., 1998). In other words, young adults completed measures about their middle-aged parents, and their middle-aged parents completed measures about their aged parents. Parental caregiving was assessed by using the Activities of Daily Living Scale (Stein et al., 1998), which assesses how frequently adults report assisting their parents with 11 activities of daily living, including activities traditionally performed by both women and men. The Filial Responsibility Composite Index, a 10-item scale composed of items commonly used by researchers in the area (Finley et al., 1988; Hanson et al., 1983), was used to assess attitudes of adult children about responsibilities to aging parents. We also used the 17-item Affection Toward Parents Measure developed by Walker and Thompson (1983) to assess intimacy with parents.

We purposely used an intergenerational rather than a cohort research design to examine how two generations of family members viewed obligation in their relationships with their parents. *Generation* refers to lineage position within families (e.g., grandparents, parents, children) and *cohort* refers to a group of individuals born at a particular point in historical time. An intergenerational approach allowed us to examine the degree of similarity as well as generational differences between parents and adult children in their reports of obligation. We felt that examining the degree of intrafamily similarity or "intergenerational transmission" (Troll & Bengtson, 1979) might be particularly important given that young adults are likely to observe their parents and grandparents interacting with each other (Watkins et al., 1987).

The sample of 230 young adults (54 men, 176 women) who participated in the research can be characterized as unmarried college undergraduates who were around 19 years old. The majority of the young adult sample lived less than a day's drive from their parents' homes and reported relatively frequent telephone and face-to-face contact with their parents. The 230 middle-aged adults (97 men, 133 women) in the study were on average about 45 years old, had graduated high school or completed some college, and had three children. More than half of the sample reported having one living parent, which was most frequently their mother, and the rest of the sample reported having both parents currently living. The sample of middle-aged parents reported that their older parents were an average of 72 years old. Similar to their adult children, a majority of the middle-aged sample reported relatively frequent contact with their parents and lived within a day's drive of their parents' homes. Adults in the study generally characterized their middle-aged and older parents as being in relatively good health.

As expected, women in both generations reported higher levels of parental caregiving, on average, than did men. Both generations of women generally felt a greater sense of obligation to maintain contact and participate in family ritual, provide assistance, avoid conflict, and engage in personal sharing with their parents than did men. Both men and women in the middle-aged sample generally reported similar levels of obligation to be self-sufficient. However, young adult women generally reported a greater sense of obligation to be self-sufficient than did young adult men. In addition, both middle-aged men and women with one living parent reported feeling a greater obligation to provide assistance than did middle-aged adults with two living parents. The lack of gender differences may suggest that circumstances of older parents play an equally important role for both daughters and sons in eliciting felt obligation to provide parental assistance.

Gender of the adult child was used in the research as a base-rate variable to describe the predictive power of felt obligation in adults' reports of parental caregiving. For both generations, felt obligation was a better predictor of adults' reports of parental caregiving than was the gender of the adult child. Results of hierarchical multiple regression analyses indicated that felt obligation scores accounted for an additional 10% of the variance in adults' reports of parental caregiving beyond that of gender in the young adult sample. In the middle-aged sample, felt obligation scores accounted for an additional 16% of the variance in reports of caregiving beyond that of gender. It appears that knowing adults' overall level of felt obligation was more useful in estimating their reports of parental caregiving than was simply knowing whether they were daughters or sons.

The study also examined the ability of felt obligation to account for variation in adults' reports of parental caregiving as compared with two well-established constructs in the caregiving literature, filial responsibility and parental affection. Here again, although filial responsibility and parental affection accounted for variance in respondents' reports of caregiving, felt obligation scores accounted for a significant amount of additional variance in both young and middle-aged adult respondents' reports. Findings suggest that when it comes to providing care, adults' feeling of obligation in the context of their ongoing relationship with their parents is more salient than feelings of affection and general attitudes about filial responsibility combined.

Intergenerational differences between young adults and their middle-aged parents in reports of felt obligation far outweighed any similarities. On average, young adults reported feeling more obligated to maintain contact and family ritual, provide assistance, avoid conflict, be self-sufficient, and engage in personal sharing in their relationships with their middle-aged parents than did middle-aged adults in their relationships with their older parents. These findings are consistent with the view of obligation as arising from feelings of indebtedness toward parents that need to be repaid (Finch, 1989; Rossi & Rossi, 1990). Middle-aged adults, in general, have greater opportunity to reciprocate with their parents than do young adults, given greater access to resources in middle age and the sheer amount of time they have spent as adults relating to their parents. The young adults in the study sample were attending college, and they might have been more dependent on their parents, at least financially, than others in their age cohort. In other words, undergraduates may have even greater feelings of indebtedness and fewer resources than adults of the same age who are employed and living independently from their parents.

WHAT ABOUT FELT OBLIGATION TOWARD PARENTS IN LATER LIFE? A PRELIMINARY LOOK

The discussion thus far has focused on the advantages of a life course perspective in the study of obligation toward parents in adulthood. Felt obligation has been described as a conceptualization of family obligation that is relational in nature; it assumes that obligation is negotiated within the context of ongoing relationships between children and parents across the life course. Felt obligation offers a more nuanced treatment of the rights and duties that accompany kin roles than attitudinal approaches to family obligation such as filial responsibility. It acknowledges the importance of social norms while being sensitive to individual negotiations about obligations between children and parents that occur in the context of family and personal history and phase of life.

The theoretical significance of felt obligation is the view that the origins of obligation lie in the sacrifices that parents make in the course of childrearing and the salience of obligation for children and parents throughout adulthood. This view is in direct contrast with attitudinal approaches, which assume that parents' infirmities and need for care are the catalysts for obligation. Empirical studies support the view that felt obligation toward parents is present in young adulthood and, in fact, has greater salience for young adults than for adults in middle age. Research has suggested the practical significance of the felt obligation construct in understanding adults' reports of parental caregiving or helping beyond that of filial responsibility and affection. Although women predominate as family caregivers, research suggests that felt obligation can account for variation in adults' reports of parental caregiving beyond that of gender of the adult child. Overall, studies highlight the promise of felt obligation as a powerful construct in research on families in adulthood.

Of course, many questions remain unanswered in the study of felt obligation between adults and their parents. Felt obligation toward parents has been investigated in early and middle adulthood, but little is known about the feelings of obligation that older adults may have toward their aged parents. Perhaps older adults have relatively low levels of felt obligation because of the continued opportunities to repay parents over the life course for parental sacrifices made in child rearing. However, it is also possible that circumstances associated with this life phase uniquely contribute to aspects of felt obligation. For example, felt obligation may increase toward aged parents, given the reality that parents will not be alive forever. The fact that adult children themselves are approaching old age may also enter into their relationships with aged parents. Feelings of obligation toward parents in later life may also become more complicated by levels of informal and formal caregiving received by parents. Would high levels of informal caregiving by adults, particularly daughters, in later life lead to lower levels of felt obligation, given that older adults would be actively involved in making sacrifices to repay aged parents? Similarly, would levels of felt obligation be lower if parents in need were receiving formal caregiving services that reduced the necessity for family care?

To begin to examine felt obligation toward parents in later life, my colleagues and I recently completed a study of 157 older adult children (99 women, 58 men) whose parents were residents of assisted living communities in the Midwest (Stein, Hunt, & Mann, 2007). We decided to study felt obligation among older adults with parents in assisted living so that level of formal caregiving to parents would be less of a complicating factor. All parents of older adults in the study were residents of assisted living communities managed by one corporation that used the same criteria for admittance to their facilities in different geographical areas. We made the simplifying assumption that the parents of older adults in our study were generally receiving the level of formal care that they needed within the assisted living community. To recruit participants for the study, adult children who were listed as primary contacts for residents of five assisted living communities across southeastern Michigan were mailed a letter that described the study. They were asked to participate in the research by completing and returning an enclosed survey regarding their relationships with their parents in assisted living. The return rate for the survey was about 55%.

A number of research questions motivated the study, but one question relevant to the present discussion concerns the role of parent characteristics in older adults' reports of felt obligation. We felt that the health status of parents might be particularly important in older adults' reports of felt obligation and hypothesized that the more infirm older adults perceived their aged parents to be, the more obligation they would report feeling toward their parents. For comparative purposes, we assessed differences in older adults' reports of filial responsibility and frequency of their contact with parents by telephone and face-to-face visits as a function of their perceptions of parents' health status. We also examined gender differences in felt obligation, frequency of contact, and filial responsibility.

Adult children in the study were around 57 years old ($SD = 7.4$), married (86%), with an average of about 3 children ($SD = 1.6$). Slightly over half (51%) of the sample were employed full time, and a quarter of the sample were retired. A total of 43% of the sample reported annual household incomes of more than $80,000, and 54% of the sample reported having completed college or obtained postgraduate degrees. A majority of adult children reported being involved or extremely involved in their parent's life (75%) and felt primarily responsible for making decisions about their parent's care (67%).

A total of 77% of adult children reported on their relationship with their mother, which included a total of 80 mother–daughter relationships and 41 mother–son relationships. There were 19 father–daughter relationships and 17 father–son ties. Aged parents were on average 86 years of age ($SD = 7.1$) and had been in the assisted living community for an average of a little more than 3 years ($M = 39$ months; $SD = 30$ months). Adults reported frequent face-to-face visits with parents; 44% of the sample reporting visiting several times a week and 36% reporting weekly visits. Frequent telephone contact with parents was also reported: 64% of the sample reported telephone contact several times a week, and 17% reported weekly phone contact.

We were particularly interested in understanding whether adults' perceptions of their parents' physical health and mental abilities were related to their reports of felt obligation. Although we asked a number of specific questions about adults' views of their parents' physical health, we also decided to include two items that asked adults to rate their aged parents' physical health and mental abilities (ability to understand and communicate, memory, etc.) with respect to other people their parents' age. Adult children responded to each item using a 5-point scale ranging from 1 = *much worse than others her (his) age* to 5 = *much better than others her (his) age*. For ease of analysis, ratings of health status were collapsed into two categories to indicate adults' perceptions of aged parents as "much better than others her (his) age" or "the same or worse than others her (his) age" for the physical health and mental abilities items. Adults also rated the frequency of face-to-face and telephone contact with their parents and completed the Filial Responsibility Composite Index to assess attitudes of adult children about responsibilities to aging parents (Stein, 1992).

We wanted to consider adults' views of both the physical health and mental abilities of their aged parents simultaneously. To do this, we divided the sample into four groups on the basis of their dichotomized ratings of their parents' physical health and mental abilities. Results of a cross-tabulation of physical health and mental abilities ratings indicate that 35% of adults viewed both the physical health and mental abilities of their parents as better than others, and 26% of adults viewed both the physical and mental abilities of parents as the same as or worse than others. A total of 22% of the sample viewed parents' physical abilities as better and mental abilities as the same as or worse than others, and 17% viewed mental abilities as better and physical health as the same as or worse than others. We can see that by characterizing adults' perceptions of both their parents' physical health and mental abilities simultaneously, almost 40% of the sample perceived discrepancies between their parents' physical health and mental abilities.

We used these four combined ratings of parents' health status (e.g., both physical and mental abilities better, both physical and mental abilities worse, physical health better and mental abilities worse, physical health worse and mental abilities better than others their age) to investigate mean differences in older adults' reports of frequency of contact with parents, filial responsibility, and felt obligation toward aged parents. Results of a series of one-way analysis of variance (ANOVA) procedures indicated no significant differences in adults' reports of face-to-face contact with parents, telephone contact with parents, or filial responsibility as a function of adults' combined ratings of parents' physical health and mental abilities.

To investigate differences in adults' reports of felt obligation as a function of parent health status, a multivariate analysis of variance was conducted using the four categories of combined ratings of health status as the independent variable and the five dimensions of felt obligation as dependent variables in the analysis. Findings indicated a significant main effect for combined health ratings, $F(15, 348) = 2.7, p = .001$. Results of the ANOVAs for each of the five felt obligation subscales indicated significant differences in respondents' scores on obligation to provide assistance, $F(3, 130) = 5.3, p < .05$; to engage in personal sharing, $F(3, 130) = 3.5, p < .05$; and to avoid conflict, $F(3, 130) = 3.2, p < .05$.

Results of post hoc comparisons of health status means using Bonferroni correction indicated that older adults who viewed their aged parents' physical health as better and their mental abilities as worse than others reported that they felt significantly more obligated to provide assistance than older adults who viewed their aged parents physical and mental abilities as better than others ($M = 4.5$ vs. $M = 3.9$, respectively). In terms of personal sharing, older adults who viewed their parents' physical health as worse and their mental abilities as better than others reported feeling significantly more obligated to engage in personal sharing than older adults whose parents were viewed as both physically and mentally better off than others ($M = 2.8$ vs. $M = 2.3$, respectively) and also reported more obligation to engage in personal sharing than respondents whose parents are viewed as both physically and mentally worse off than others ($M = 2.8$ vs. $M = 2.2$, respectively). After controlling for multiple comparisons, no significant differences in respondents' scores on obligation to avoid conflict were found as a function of health status.

To summarize, significant differences in felt obligation were reported among older adults who perceived a discrepancy between their aged parents' physical health and mental abilities. Specifically, adults who perceived their parents' physical health as better and their mental abilities as worse than others reported significantly more obligation to assist their parents than those adults viewing both aspects of their parents health status as better than others. Moreover, adults who viewed their parents' mental abilities as better than others and their physical health as worse reported more obligation to share personal information with parents than those who perceived both their parents' health and mental abilities positively or both aspects of their parents' health status negatively.

These findings suggest that it is the discrepancies in adults' view of their parents' physical health and mental abilities that contribute to feelings of obligation in specific domains. It may be that when older adults feel that their aged parents are doing better mentally and less well physically, they feel obligated to focus on parents' cognitive strengths by engaging in more personal sharing with their parents. In contrast, when adult children perceive aged parents as doing less well mentally and better physically, they feel obligated to provide direct assistance, regardless of the fact that parents reside in assisted living communities.

In terms of gender, both adult daughters and sons in the study reported similar levels of filial responsibility, frequency of contact, and feelings of obligation toward aged parents. Note that the sample consisted of older adults identified as primary contacts for their parents in the assisted living communities. This sample selection bias may account for the lack of gender differences in the study. In other words, sons who have chosen to take primary responsibility for their parents appear to respond no differently than daughters in their reports of felt obligation, filial responsibility, and frequency of interactions with aged parents. Of course, research that compares felt obligation of older adults whose aged parents are in assisted living with older adults whose parents live independently is needed to replicate and extend present findings.

RESEARCHING FELT OBLIGATION TOWARD PARENTS: CURRENT LIMITATIONS AND FUTURE DIRECTIONS

Although research on felt obligation has generated a number of important and intriguing findings, existing studies are limited in several respects. Findings are based on relatively small, nonrandom samples of primarily

Caucasian adults living in the midwestern United States. To date, only one study has examined differences in felt obligation as a function of ethnicity (Freeberg & Stein, 1996). Studies use cross-sectional research designs to provide "snapshots" of adults' reports of relationships with parents at one point in time. Existing studies examine felt obligation for both men and women, but men are still underrepresented in study samples. Studies have been conducted primarily with intact families, and the role of felt obligation toward parents in different family structures remains unexamined. Larger, more representative, and diverse samples are needed to understand the generalizability of the felt obligation construct and to further examine similarities and differences in felt obligation as a function of ethnicity, socioeconomic status, geographical location, family structure, and gender. Although studies suggest differences in felt obligation toward parents at different periods in the life course, longitudinal research is needed to examine how adults negotiate felt obligation toward parents in the context of family relationships that grow and change over time.

In future research, the meaning and implications of felt obligation in adult–parent relationships can be investigated at a variety of levels. A central focus of our research has been on issues of stability and change in felt obligation toward parents across the adult life course. Previous studies have demonstrated the importance of felt obligation toward parents in young and middle adulthood, and preliminary findings reported here also suggest that felt obligation toward parents may also be meaningful in later life. A cohort study that compares adults' reports of felt obligation toward parents in young, middle, and later adulthood would be a valuable next step in describing felt obligation across the life course.

Previous studies of felt obligation have been conducted exclusively from the perspective of the individual. Multiple perspectives research would deepen our understanding of the salience of felt obligation from the perspective of both adults and their parents and may provide insight into how aspects of obligation are negotiated between adults and parents across time. Qualitative research methods may be particularly useful in understanding the subtleties involved in the negotiation of felt obligation at the dyadic level, as adults and parents may have their own language for describing the rights and duties that they perceive in their relationships.

Qualitative studies of felt obligation from multiple perspectives would allow us to examine the level of consensus between adults and parents about perceived obligations and how consensus might affect other aspects of adult–parent ties. Multiple perspectives research might also shed additional light on felt obligation as a motive for helping, both for adults and parents. Although gerontologists focus primarily on adults' caregiving to aged parents, research suggests that the direction of helping exchanges between adults and their parents is primarily from parents to children through most of the adult life course (Spitze & Logan, 1992). Little is known about felt obligation of parents to children as a motive for parents' providing help to their children in adulthood.

Felt obligation should also be investigated within the context of family history. Evidence suggests that daughters who live in close geographical proximity to parents are most likely to be caregivers to them (Spitze & Logan, 1992), but relatively little is known about the process of "nomination" or "negotiation" among siblings about who will take primary responsibility for parents' care. It is unclear whether felt obligation toward parents differs among siblings and how felt obligation might contribute to siblings' role in parental helping. Family circumstances (e.g., divorce) or various family structures (e.g., blended or single-parent families) are also likely to affect adults' feelings of obligation. The role of family structure and family history in adults' feelings of parental obligation and the implications for individual well-being are important directions for future research.

A feminist perspective encourages further analysis of the role of felt obligation at the social systems level as a source of oppression for women. The family is a major context for socialization, where family members construct and perpetuate beliefs about who does what within the family and in the larger world. Our first lessons about dominant social hierarchies, which shape our experience of gender, race, and social class, are typically learned within the family. Felt obligation toward parents may help perpetuate the belief that women have a responsibility to sacrifice their own needs and desires to serve the needs of others (Gilligan, 1982; Miller, 1986). As Baber and Allen (1992) noted, the oppression of women results from beliefs, attitudes, and acts that exclude women in general from access to resources, power, and opportunities for personal growth and development. Gendered relations within the family help develop and sustain the complex system of structures, processes, and relationships that perpetuate women's oppression. Feminist scholars articulate a major paradox in transforming gender relations within families in ways that do not perpetuate social oppression. It is a fact that for many women, the very aspects of family life that serve to oppress them also offer opportunities for personal validation, agency, and fulfillment. Much work is needed to understand the major personal and social consequences of felt obligation toward parents in adulthood.

REFERENCES

Abel, E. (1989). Family care of the frail elderly. In E. Abel & M. Nelson (Eds.), *Circles of care: Work and identity in women's lives* (pp. 65–91). Albany: SUNY Press.

Abel, E., & Nelson, M. (1990). Circles of care: An introductory essay. In E. Abel & M. Nelson (Eds.), *Circles of care: Work and identity in women's lives* (pp. 4–34). Albany: SUNY Press.

Adams, B. N. (1968). *Kinship in an urban setting.* Chicago: Markham.

Alwin, D. F. (1995). Taking time seriously: Studying social change, social structure and human lives. In P. Moen, G. H. Elder Jr., & K. Luscher (Eds.), *Examining lives in context: Perspectives on the ecology of human development* (pp. 211–262). Washington, DC: American Psychological Association.

Baber, K. M., & Allen, K. R. (1992). *Women and families: Feminist reconstructions.* New York: Guilford Press.

Bahr, H. M. (1976). The kinship role. In F. I. Nye (Ed.), *Role structure and analysis of the family* (pp. 61–80). Beverly Hills, CA: Sage.

Blieszner, R., & Mancini, J. (1987). Enduring ties: Older adults' parental role and responsibilities. *Family Relations, 36,* 176–180.

Cicirelli, V. G. (1993). Attachment and obligation as daughters' motives for caregiving behavior and subsequent effect of subjective burden. *Psychology and Aging, 8,* 144–155.

Coward, R., & Dwyer, J. (1990). The association of gender, sibling network composition, and patterns of parent care by adult children. *Research on Aging, 12,* 158–181.

Di Leonardo, M. (1987). The female world of cards and holidays: Women, families, and the work of kinship. *Signs, 12,* 440–453.

Finch, J. (1989). *Family obligation and social change.* Cambridge, MA: Policy Press.

Finley, N. J., Roberts, D., & Banahan, B. F. (1988). Motivators and inhibitors of attitudes of filial obligation toward aging parents. *The Gerontologist, 28*, 73–78.

Freeberg, A. L., & Stein, C. H. (1996). Felt obligation towards parents in Mexican-American and Anglo-American young adults. *Journal of Social and Personal Relationships, 13*, 457–471.

Gelfand, D. E. (1989). Immigration, aging, and intergenerational relationships. *The Gerontologist, 29*, 366–372.

Gilligan, C. (1982). *In a different voice.* Cambridge, MA: Harvard University Press.

Graham, H. (1985). Providers, negotiators and mediators: Women as hidden carers. In E. Lewin & V. Oleson (Eds.), *Women, health and healing* (pp. 25–52). London: Tavistock.

Greenfield, E. A., & Marks, N. F. (2006). Linked lives: Adult children's problems and their parents' psychological and relational well-being. *Journal of Marriage and Family, 68*, 442–454.

Hagestad, G. O. (1991). The aging society as a context for family life. In Nancy S. Jedler (Ed.), *Aging and ethics* (pp. 123–146). Tobowa, NJ: Humana Press.

Hagestad, G. O. (1996). On-time, off-time, out of time? Reflections on continuity and discontinuity from an illness process. In V. L. Bengtson (Ed.), *Adulthood and aging: Research on continuities and discontinuities: A tribute to Bernice Neugarten* (pp. 204–222). New York: Springer Publishing Company.

Hagestad, G. O., & Neugarten, B. (1985). Age and the life course. In R. Binstock & E. Shanas (Eds.), *The handbook of aging and society* (2nd ed., pp. 35–61). New York: Van Nostrand-Reinhold.

Hamon, R. R., & Blieszner, R. (1990). Filial responsibility expectations among adult child–older parent pairs. *Journal of Gerontology: Psychological Sciences, 45*, 110–112.

Hanson, S. L., Sauer, W. J., & Seelbach, W. C. (1983). Racial and cohort variations in filial responsibility norms. *The Gerontologist, 23*, 626–631.

Hareven, T. K. (1986). American families in transition: Historical perspectives on change. In A. S. Skolnick & J. H. Skolnick (Eds.), *Family in transition* (pp. 40–58). Boston: Little, Brown.

Hareven, T. K. (1991). Synchronizing individual time, family time, and historical time. In J. Bender & D. E. Wellbery (Eds.), *Chronotypes: The construction of time* (pp. 167–182). Palo Alto, CA: Stanford University Press

Hochschild, A. (1989). *The second shift: Working parents and the revolution at home.* New York: Viking Penguin.

Hooyman, N. R., & Gonyea, J. (1995). *Feminist perspectives on family care: Polices for gender justice.* Thousand Oaks, CA: Sage.

Horowitz, A. (1985). Sons and daughters and caregivers to older parents: Differences in role performance and consequences. *The Gerontologist, 25*, 612–617.

Jarrett, W. H. (1985). Caregiving within kinship systems: Is affection really necessary? *The Gerontologist, 25,* 5–10.

Karpel, M. A., & Strauss, E. S. (1983). *Family evaluation.* New York: Gardner Press.

Laditka, J. N., & Laditka, S. B. (2001). Adult children helping older parents. *Research on Aging, 23,* 429–456.

Matthews, S. H., & Rosner, T. T. (1988). Shared filial responsibility: The family as the primary caregiver. *Journal of Marriage and the Family, 50,* 185–195.

McGraw, L. A., & Walker, A. J. (2004). Negotiation care: Ties between aging mothers and their caregiving daughters. *Journal of Gerontology: Social Sciences, 59B,* S324–S352.

Miller, J. B. (1986). *Toward a new psychology of women* (2nd ed.). Boston: Beacon.

Quinn, W. H. (1983). Personal and family adjustment in later life. *Journal of Marriage and the Family, 45,* 57–73.

Rappaport, J. (1995). Empowerment meets narrative: Listening to stories and creating settings. *American Journal of Community Psychology, 23,* 795–807.

Reiss, P. J. (1962). The extended kinship system: Correlates of and attitudes on frequency of interaction. *Marriage and Family Living, 27,* 333–339.

Rindfuss, R., Swicegood, C., & Rosenfeld, R. (1987). Disorder in the life course: How common and does it matter? *American Sociological Review, 52,* 785–801.

Rossi, A. S., & Rossi, P. H. (1990). *Of human bonding: Parent–child relations across the life course.* New York: Aldine de Gruyter.

Schorr, A. (1980). " . . . *thy father & thy mother . . . ": A second look at filial responsibility and family policy.* Washington, DC: U.S. Department of Health and Human Services, U.S. Government Printing Office.

Seelbach, W. C. (1984). Filial responsibility and the care of aging family members. In W. H. Quinn & G. A. Hughston (Eds.), *Independent aging: Family and social systems perspectives* (pp. 92–105). Rockville, MD: Aspen.

Seelbach, W. C., & Sauer, W. J. (1977). Filial responsibility and morale among aged parents. *The Gerontologist, 17,* 492–499.

Settersten, R. A. (2003). Propositions and controversies in life-course scholarship. In R. A. Settersten (Ed.), *Invitation to the life course: Toward new understandings of later life* (pp. 15–48). Amityville, NY: Baywood.

Settersten, R. A., & Hagestad, G. O. (1996). What's the latest? Cultural age deadlines for family transitions. *The Gerontologist, 36,* 178–188.

Spitze, G., & Logan, J. R. (1990). Sons, daughters, and intergenerational social support. *Journal of Marriage and the Family, 52,* 420–430.

Spitze, G., & Logan, J. R. (1992). Helping as a component of parent–adult child relations. *Research on Aging, 14,* 291–312.

Stein, C. H. (1992). Ties that bind: Three studies of obligation in adult relationships with family. *Journal of Social and Personal Relationships, 9,* 525–547.

Stein, C. H. (1993). Felt obligation in adult family relationships. In S. Duck (Ed.), *Social context and relationships* (pp. 78–99). Newbury Park, CA: Sage.

Stein, C. H., Hunt, M. G., & Mann, L. M. (2007). *Felt obligation of older adults towards their aged parents: Adults' perceptions of parents' physical health and mental abilities.* Manuscript in preparation.

Stein, C. H., & Rappaport, J. (1986). Social network interviews as sources of etic and emic data: A study of young married women. In S. E. Hobfoll (Ed.), *Stress, social support and women* (pp. 47–66). New York: Hemisphere.

Stein, C. H., & Ward, M. (1997). *Felt obligation enactment and individual psychological well being correlates in non-distressed married couples.* Unpublished manuscript.

Stein, C. H., & Wemmerus, V. A. (2001). Searching for a normal life: Personal accounts of adults with schizophrenia, their parents and well-siblings. *American Journal of Community Psychology, 29,* 725–746.

Stein, C. H., Wemmerus, V. A., Ward, M., Gaines, M. E., Freeberg, A. L., & Jewell, T. C. (1998). Because they're my parents: An intergenerational study of felt obligation and parental caregiving. *Journal of Marriage and the Family, 60,* 611–622.

Stoller, E. P. (1990). Males as helpers: The role of sons, relatives and friends. *The Gerontologist, 30,* 226–235.

Stoller, E. P. (1994). Teaching about gender: The experience of family care of frail elderly relatives. *Educational Gerontology, 20,* 679–697.

Traustadottir, R. (1991). Mothers who care: Gender, disability, and family life. *Journal of Family Issues, 12,* 211–228.

Troll, L. E., & Bengtson, V. (1979). Generations in the family. In W. R. Burr, F. I. Nye, R. Hill, & I. L. Reiss (Eds.), *Contemporary theories about the family* (pp. 127–161). New York: Free Press.

Walker, A. (1992). Conceptual perspectives on gender and family caregiving. In J. Dwyer & R. Coward (Eds.), *Gender, families and elder care.* (pp. 34–48). Newbury Park, CA: Sage.

Walker, A. J., Pratt, C. C., Shinn, H., & Jones, L. L. (1990). Motives for parental caregiving and relationship quality. *Family Relations, 39,* 51–56.

Walker, A. J., & Thompson, L. (1983). Intimacy and intergenerational aid and contact among mothers and daughters *Journal of Marriage and the Family, 45,* 841–849.

Watkins, S. C., Menken, J. A., & Bongaarts, J. (1987). Demographic foundations of family change. *American Sociological Review, 52,* 346–358.

5

Women at Midlife: Stress and Rewards of Balancing Parent Care With Employment and Other Family Roles

Mary Ann Parris Stephens, Melissa M. Franks,
Lynn M. Martire, Tina R. Norton, and Audie A. Atienza

Within the life span development framework, it is important to understand that development is dependent on history. This is evident
when discussing middle adulthood. "Midlife" is a relatively new social construction in the United States and other Western countries (Etaugh &
Bridges, 2006) and has come about through a variety of societal changes that
accelerated during the 20th century, including better overall health and
greater longevity. These trends have increased opportunities for women to
enjoy active and productive careers and personal lives beyond their childbearing and child-rearing years and at the same time have increased the
probability that women will have aging parents who will develop chronic
and disabling health conditions. In this chapter, we explore whether emerging opportunities in women's work and family lives at this stage of life may
benefit their well-being through strengthening their resilience in managing
their multiple roles, particularly the care of an aging parent.

This chapter focuses on women who are attempting to balance their
parent-care responsibilities with the challenges of their mother, wife, and
employee roles. We first examine sociodemographic characteristics of
these women and life course perspectives on adult development, families,
and later life caregiving. Next, we review theoretical and empirical literature that bears on the experiences of women in multiple roles that

include parent care. Our review highlights the programmatic research that we and our colleagues have conducted since the early 1990s. We end this chapter with a discussion of social policies that affect women in midlife, including implications of our work for women attempting to balance multiple roles.

WOMEN AT MIDLIFE
AND CHANGING DEMOGRAPHIC TRENDS

Although the term *midlife* is often used to refer to the period of life somewhere between the ages of 40 and 60, this phase of life is not easily defined by age. Middle adulthood for women may better be characterized by a constellation of common life events and developments, including biological changes, children leaving home, and becoming a grandparent (Etaugh & Bridges, 2006). For most women, this time in life is one of zest, personal growth, and enjoyment of freedom from childbearing and responsibilities for young children (Mitchell & Helson, 1990). At the same time, however, many women in midlife take on new family roles and responsibilities when aging parents or parents-in-law become ill and need their assistance.

Since the early 1980s, researchers have paid a great deal of attention to midlife women who provide parent care and simultaneously occupy other family and work roles. These women have often been referred to as "women in the middle" (Brody, 1981). This label can refer to the generational position of these women, in that they are between the older generation of their parents and the younger generation of children. It also can refer to their chronological age in that these women are in the middle years of the life span (Brody, 1990).

Although awareness of women in the middle began more than 25 years ago, the issues and concerns raised at that time appear to be even more applicable to today's women and those who will enter midlife in the near future. Within the framework of life span development, the role of history is evident from the large cohort of babies born in the 2 decades following World War II (*baby boomers*) who are now in their parent-care years. The parents of these individuals are living longer than any generation in history, and women in the baby boomer cohort are postponing childbearing later into adulthood and continue to participate in the paid labor force at record levels. According to census data, one half of American women in their middle years are married and are in the paid labor force, and more than one third are married and have a child under the age of 18 (U.S. Bureau of the Census, 2006). Therefore, today's midlife women are more in the middle than ever before (Brody, 2004).

Increased longevity has brought with it many dramatic societal changes, not the least of which is the rapidly swelling number of adults who will need care and support in their later years. During the 1990s, significant changes emerged in the demography of later life caregiving in the United States (Wolff & Kasper, 2006). The proportion of adult child primary caregivers was 41.3% in 1999, an increase from 35.9% in 1989. During the same decade, the proportion of care recipients receiving help with only instrumental activities of daily living (ADLs) decreased, whereas the proportion receiving help with five or more personal ADLs increased. Consistent with the trend for more adult children to assume the parent-care role and for older adults to be in poorer health, the proportion of caregivers providing help on a daily basis increased substantially between 1989 and 1999, and this change was most notable among adult child caregivers.

The *parent support ratio*—number of adults 85 and older per 100 adults aged 50 to 64—is another index of changing demographic trends in American families. This ratio suggests the potential for how many middle-aged persons are supporting the oldest old. Individuals making up the middle-aged group are often children of the very old, hence the use of the term *parent*. In 2000, the parent support ratio in the United States was 10; that is, for every 100 midlife adults there were 10 older family members to attend to, a threefold increase from 3 older family members for every 100 midlife adults in 1960. This ratio is projected to climb to 16 by 2030 and to continue to rise to 30 by 2050—when all baby boomers themselves will be aged 85 and older (He, Sengupta, Velkoff, & DeBarros, 2005). If these forecasts are correct, the parent support ratio will triple in only a half century, and thus increasing numbers of middle-aged adults are likely to enter the parent-care role.

Although men increased slightly in representation among adult child caregivers during the 1990s, this role remains highly gendered, with almost three quarters of all adult child caregivers in 1999 being women (Wolff & Kasper, 2006). The average caregiver in the United States is a woman who is 46 years of age, married, and works outside the home earning an annual income of $35,000. Although men also provide caregiving assistance, female caregivers spend as much as 50% more time providing care than their male counterparts (MetLife Mature Market Institute, National Alliance for Caregiving, & The National Center on Women and Aging, 1999).

Early research on women in the middle estimated that in addition to having the roles of mother, wife, and employee, 14% of women between the ages of 40 and 69 also have at least one living parent (Rosenthal, Matthews, & Marshall, 1989). Other research has estimated that 14% of women ages 40 to 64 provide at least 3 hours of assistance per week to a parent, and 4% provide that much assistance to a parent-in-law (Spitze & Logan, 1990). Moreover, the likelihood of being in the role of family caregiver has been shown to increase both with age and across birth cohorts (Moen, Robinson, & Fields, 1994), suggesting that many more women will occupy the parent-care role in the future.

Because so many adult daughters provide parent care, some have argued that parent care is becoming a normative experience in American families, and that these women find themselves increasingly caught between the competing demands of their multiple family and work roles (Brody, 1985). This trend also has been widely publicized in the popular media. Such claims initially sparked academic debate about how common it is for women to simultaneously occupy the parent-care, mother, wife, and employee roles (e.g., Boyd & Treas, 1989; Spitze & Logan, 1990). Gerontologists have agreed, however, that even though multiple role configurations that include the parent-care role may not be normative (in the sense of characterizing a majority of middle-aged women), an increasingly large number of women are faced with these multiple role responsibilities, and this trend is likely to continue into the foreseeable future.

At this historical nexus, we and our colleagues began our work with women in the middle. In the following sections, we highlight our key findings on the health effects of role constellations that combine parent care with various family and work roles. Before doing so, however, we describe the theoretical underpinnings of this work.

THEORETICAL PERSPECTIVES ON WOMEN'S MULTIPLE ROLES

The *competing demands hypothesis* evolved to explain the negative effects that caregiving often has on caregivers' psychological and physical well-being. This perspective argues that multiple role responsibilities create demands on women that compete for their time and energy. The competing demands hypothesis rests on assumptions similar to those of the *scarcity hypothesis*, which assumes that individuals have limited personal resources and that social organizations and role partners demand all of these resources (Goode, 1960). Thus, an individual's total role obligations are thought to be overly demanding, making role conflict inevitable.

The scarcity hypothesis has been challenged by the *expansion hypothesis*, which emphasizes the energy gains, rather than the energy expenditures, accrued by individuals with multiple roles (Marks, 1977). This energy-expansion perspective predicts positive consequences resulting from the enhancement of such personal resources as mastery, self-esteem, identity, and social and material gains from various roles. Moreover, when resources are scarce in one role, it is assumed that resources are likely to be available from other roles to compensate. Indeed, a growing literature on women's health has shown that occupying multiple roles (most often those of mother, wife, and employee) is associated with better overall well-being (e.g., Ahrens & Ryff, 2006; Waldron & Jacobs, 1989).

Although the scarcity and expansion perspectives make different predictions about the effects of multiple roles, both are limited in that they focus on the number of roles occupied rather than on the quality of experiences that transpire within roles. Both perspectives, with their emphasis on quantity, predict a net gain or a net loss of resources regardless of role experiences. In contrast, perspectives that emphasize the quality of role experiences assert that two similar roles could create different cost–benefit ratios within and across these roles. The role quality perspective asserts that both problems and rewards experienced within a role should be considered (Barnett & Baruch, 1985).

Drawing from prior work emphasizing role quality over role occupancy, our research with adult daughter caregivers has been largely driven by two opposing questions: Do the roles that these women occupy in addition to the parent-care role have deleterious effects on their well-being (as the competing demands perspective assumes) or do these additional roles benefit their well-being (as the expansion perspective assumes)? Our work also has been guided by a third intriguing question: Are some roles more psychologically central (personally important) to women than others? To address these questions, we conducted a series of studies in which we conceptualized the parent-care role as an important family role that women experience as a part of their larger family and work life.

PARENT CARE AND OTHER FAMILY ROLES

At the time we began our work, caregiving research had largely overlooked issues of role quality. This research typically focused on the problems associated with parent care and had given little attention to the positive aspects of care provision. Moreover, this work tended to examine the caregiver role in isolation from other roles. When other roles were considered, they often were not given weight equal to that of the caregiver role. In our studies of family roles, we focused on women who occupied not only the role of caregiver to a parent or parent-in-law (i.e., primary family member who provided ADL assistance) but also the roles of wife and of mother to children at home.

Evidence for the Competing Demands Hypothesis

Guided by the competing demands hypothesis, we set out to identify sources of stress and conflict in women's family roles as well as the effects of these problems on women's psychological well-being. In the parent-care role, women most often report stressors such as the interpersonal conflict they experience when the parent criticizes or complains or is unresponsive, uncooperative, or demanding. These women also experience stress in each of their additional roles as mothers and wives. In the mother role, the stressors most often mentioned are the heavy demands of or responsibilities for children, arguments with children, uncertainty about child-rearing practices, and the financial burdens of raising a family. Lack of companionship and emotional support from the husband and poor communication or conflict about the children are the stressors most often mentioned in the wife role. Consistent with the competing demands hypothesis, stress in these other family roles detracts from women's well-being beyond the negative effects of stress in the parent-care role (Stephens, Franks, & Townsend, 1994).

In addition to more global aspects of well-being, our work further reveals that stress in these family roles has the potential to erode women's sense of mastery. Women who experience more stress in the parent-care, mother, and wife roles also feel less confidence and competence to fulfill their responsibilities in each role domain (Franks & Stephens, 1992). Moreover, as stress increases in parent-care and mother roles over time, women's feelings of role-specific mastery continues to decline (Norton, Gupta, Stephens, Martire, & Townsend, 2005).

Our work has examined the effects of combining women's roles as mother and wife with their parent-care responsibilities (Stephens & Townsend, 1997). Our aims have been to investigate whether the stress experienced in these additional family roles might exacerbate (increase) the negative effects of parent-care stress on well-being (competing demands hypothesis) and whether the rewards experienced in these additional roles might buffer (decrease) the stress effects of parent care (expansion hypothesis). We found clear evidence to support the stress exacerbation prediction in the mother role. Parent-care stress relates to poorer well-being among women whose mother role is highly stressful, but for women whose mother role is less stressful, parent-care stress is unrelated to their well-being. In contrast, the rewards of being a mother do not appear to buffer the harmful effects of parent-care stress on well-being. Experiences in the wife role neither exacerbate nor buffer the effects of parent-care stress.

Our research team has also investigated the possibility that the experiences associated with any given role may not necessarily be confined to that role domain. Rather, because the boundaries between roles are sometimes ambiguous, it is likely that experiences in one role will spill over and color experiences in another. Role spillover is thought to be bidirectional in that experiences in one role have the potential to influence experiences in a second role and vice versa.

In our work on role spillover, we have investigated ways in which parent care and marriage might affect one another (Stephens & Franks, 1995). Consistent with competing demands, we have conceptualized *negative spillover* as the pressures on time and energy in one role that influence the quality of experiences in the other role as well as psychological interference between the roles. The type of negative spillover between the parent-care and wife roles most frequently encountered by women is the limited time available for the husband because of caregiving responsibilities. With regard to negative spillover in the other direction, very few women indicate that their marriage interferes with their parent-care responsibilities.

Evidence for the Expansion Hypothesis

Our work has been strongly influenced by assumptions of role quality perspectives, in addition to those of the expansion hypothesis. Specifically, we have assumed that to understand women's psychological well-being, it is crucial to consider the positive aspects of their multiple roles as well as the more problematic aspects. Thus, we initially identified the rewarding and satisfying features of the parent-care, mother, and wife roles.

Frequent rewards in parent care result from the satisfaction taken from knowing that their parent is well cared for, that this role fulfills a family obligation, and that they spend more time with their parent as a result of the needed assistance. As in their parent-care role, women experience many rewards as mothers and wives. As mothers, women most often find the meaning and purpose children bring to their lives to be rewarding, as well as the feeling of being needed and loved by their children. Rewards derived from being a wife most often include the husband being a good father and provider and the husband lending support and providing companionship (Stephens et al., 1994).

As predicted by the expansion hypothesis, rewards in each of these family roles contribute to psychological well-being regardless of the amount of stress occurring in each role. Moreover, an increase in rewarding experiences in the parent-care, mother, and wife roles over time tends to be accompanied by an increased sense of mastery in these roles. In fact, when increases in rewards and increases in stress are considered simultaneously, only role rewards relate to changes in mastery (Norton et al., 2005).

We also have considered ways in which these roles might benefit one another. Consistent with the role expansion hypothesis, we conceptualized *positive spillover* as involving feelings of attachment, mastery, and self-esteem in one role that influence the quality of experience in the other role. The spillover of self-esteem from one role to another is the most frequent type of positive spillover occurring in both directions. In contrast to the relative absence of negative spillover from the wife role to parent care, many women indicate that their marriage helps to bolster their parent-care experiences. Our findings reveal that both roles have the potential to foster women's feelings of self-worth and that these feelings contribute to their psychological well-being (Stephens & Franks, 1995).

Social support from the husband is yet another resource from being married that helps to offset the stress of parent care (Franks & Stephens, 1996). Women frequently receive assistance from their husbands that affords them additional time and energy to care for the parent. Moreover, some husbands provide care directly to the ill parent as a way to support their caregiving wives.

PARENT CARE AND EMPLOYMENT

Because the past several decades have witnessed increasingly large numbers of midlife women in the workforce, gerontologists have speculated about the impact of this trend. In particular, concerns have been raised about how employment will affect women's involvement in family caregiving and the long-term care of frail older adults. National data indicate that approximately half of adult children who assume the parent-care role are also employed full or part time (Wolff & Kasper, 2006).

Life course research shows that employed women are likely to continue participation in the workforce regardless of their caregiving responsibilities (Moen et al., 1994). Employed women who make the transition into family caregiving typically experience a decline in physical and mental health. Although physical limitations often attenuate with time, psychological distress accumulates over the course of care. Despite these increases in distress, however, women generally do not make changes in caregiving arrangements (Pavalko & Woodbury, 2000).

Researchers have given much attention to the health effects of employment for women (regardless of their caregiving status). Compared with those who are not employed, employed women tend to be less psychologically distressed and have better physical health and higher self-esteem (e.g., Ross & Mirowsky, 1995). So, too, the literature on later life caregiving has shown the benefits of employment for caregivers. Employed caregivers tend to experience better well-being than those who are not employed (Giele, Mutschler, & Orodenker, 1987; Miller, 1989; Skaff & Pearlin, 1992; Stoller & Pugliesi, 1989).

Because these studies of employed caregivers focused only on the occupancy of the employment role, they did not offer insight into the characteristics of women's work experiences that might be responsible for these effects. Our research team set out to fill this gap in the literature by investigating features of women's employment and work life that seemed to protect them from the harmful consequences of parent-care stress. As with our studies of caregivers' other family roles, our research on employed caregivers was guided largely by the competing demands and expansion hypotheses. That is, we were open to the possibility that occupying the dual roles of parent-care provider and employee could have both detrimental and beneficial effects on women's well-being.

Evidence for the Competing Demands Hypothesis

Studies of employed caregivers have consistently shown that the demands of parent care and employment frequently interfere with one another (e.g., Aneshensel, Pearlin, Mullan, Zarit, & Whitlatch, 1995; Gignac, Kelloway, & Gottlieb, 1996; Neal, Chapman, Ingersoll-Dayton, & Emlen, 1993) as the competing demands hypothesis predicts. Approximately half of employed primary caregivers have reported that they experience work conflict in terms of rearranging work schedules, working fewer hours, or taking time off without pay (Wolff & Kasper, 2006).

Our studies of adult daughter caregivers, all of whom were employed, married, and had children at home, have reported similar findings. When considering their other roles (mother, wife, and employee) the largest proportion of women identify the employee role as the one that conflicts most with parent care (Stephens, Townsend, Martire, & Druley, 2001).

Even though many women in our studies were employed in managerial or professional occupations, they spent an average of 3 hours per day assisting with caregiving tasks (Stephens et al., 2001). These women indicated that because of the responsibilities in these two roles, substantial conflict occurred. Women emphasized, as the competing demands hypothesis predicts, that there was not enough time and energy to do everything, the two roles were emotionally draining, and both roles imposed considerable demands on them.

In addition to investigating the conflict that often occurs at the intersection of parent care and employment, we have been interested in ways the expenditure of resources in one role might spill over to affect the other role (Stephens, Franks, & Atienza, 1997). We considered the possibility that not only may caregiving interfere with work, but work may interfere with caregiving. Being exhausted and unable to concentrate at work and having work disrupted are the interferences from parent care that women report most often. Likewise, employment frequently interferes with the amount of time and attention that women can devote to parent care. Regardless of the source of the spillover, however, we have strong evidence that the more one role interferes with functioning in another, the more likely it is that women's well-being will suffer.

Our work also suggests that the stresses of parent care and employment exert their deleterious effects on well-being through the incompatible pressures of these roles (Stephens et al., 1997). Thus, the proliferation of stressful experiences across roles appears to be one means by which stress that is specific to a given role has consequences for more global aspects of well-being. Our interrole conflict and role spillover findings are consistent with the most basic assumptions of the competing demands hypothesis, namely, that the demands of multiple roles are necessarily incompatible and can have harmful effects on well-being.

In addition to our focus on the incompatible demands of work and parent care, we have examined the possibility that the social environment of the workplace might bear on women's ability to juggle parent care and employment. Working caregivers often state that their supervisors and coworkers are sometimes insensitive about attempts to balance parent care and work or fail to understand the difficulties of providing parent care (Atienza & Stephens, 2000). Women who encounter more of such problematic interactions with their work associates also experience poorer well-being, even after considering the number of hours they work per week and the stress they experience in parent care and employment. In contrast, emotionally supportive interactions with work associates about juggling the responsibilities of parent care and work do not seem to relate to women's well-being.

Evidence for the Expansion Hypothesis

In addition to examining the resources expended in parent care and employment, our studies of employed daughter caregivers examined the resources gained from holding these dual roles, a key assumption of the expansion hypothesis. We found that as with family roles, positive experiences in the caregiver role often spill over to affect employment and vice versa (Stephens et al., 1997). Being in a good mood in one role because of rewarding experiences in the other role occurs frequently for these women. They indicate that the feelings of confidence and accomplishment they gain in one role have benefits for their other role. Although the majority of women indicate experiencing positive spillover in both directions, only spillover from the employment role to parent care relates to better well-being.

A key goal of our research team has been to identify characteristics of employment that might moderate the deleterious health effects of parent-care stress. In addition to the expansion perspective, the literature on work and women's health helped to guide this endeavor. Our studies have identified two factors that seem to function as buffers to the stress of parent care—job satisfaction and full-time employment.

As with the more general literature on women's health (e.g., Barnett & Marshall, 1992), our research has found buffering effects of rewarding employment for adult daughter caregivers (Stephens & Townsend, 1997).

Among women with less rewarding work, parent-care stress is likely to erode well-being, whereas among women with very rewarding work, parent-care stress is unlikely to be related to well-being. It is possible that women with satisfying employment are more effective in distracting themselves at work from the demands of parent care. In addition, they may be better able to regain from work such personal resources as self-esteem and mastery that are often eroded by the stress of parent care, as predicted by the expansion hypothesis.

Research on women's health has also shown that full-time employment is particularly beneficial. Working full time is associated with better well-being than is part-time employment (e.g., Wethington & Kessler, 1989). Moreover, caregivers who work more than 20 hours per week experience less stress from caregiving than those who work fewer hours (Enright & Friss, 1987). Consistent with these findings, our research has shown that among daughter caregivers who work part time, as the stress of their parent-care responsibilities increases, their well-being declines (Martire, Stephens, & Atienza, 1997). In contrast, among those working full time, no association has been shown between caregiving stress and well-being. These associations emerge even after considering work stress, the degree of the ill parents' impairment, hours of care provided, and hours of formal (paid) caregiving assistance received.

Time spent at work has the potential to provide women with much-needed respite or distraction from the responsibilities of caregiving (Brody, 1990). Thus, the stress-buffering effects of full-time employment may be due in part to the greater amount of time away from caregiving that working full time affords. The advantage of full-time work may also stem from the greater financial, social, and psychological resources it provides over part-time work.

CENTRALITY OF WOMEN'S ROLES

We next turn attention to our investigations of the personal importance that midlife women attribute to their various work and family roles, including parent care. The personal importance (centrality) of a role is thought to reflect the degree to which that role serves as an *identity anchor*, or as a means of defining one's self. Role theories have assumed that individuals gain more meaning, purpose, and behavioral guidance as a result of enacting roles that are more central to their self-concept. It is further assumed that such gains contribute to the enhancement of psychological well-being (Thoits, 1992).

Our work provides ample evidence to support these assertions in the context of women's multiple roles (Martire, Stephens, & Townsend, 2000). Adult daughters who appraise their parent-care role as being highly important also experience better well-being. A similar and even stronger pattern emerges among women for whom the mother, wife, and employee roles are judged to be highly important.

Our studies have shown that over time, the centrality of the mother and wife roles tends not to change appreciably for most women. By contrast, the centrality of the parent-care and employee roles fluctuates considerably (Norton, Stephens, Martire, Townsend, & Gupta, 2002). Whereas many women downgrade the importance of their role as parent-care provider, for some women, this role can grow in personal importance. In contrast, women are more likely to downgrade the importance of their employment over time than to amplify its importance or to view its importance as unchanged. Most notably, when considered simultaneously, role rewards are more strongly and consistently related to change in the centrality of a role than is role stress.

CONCLUSIONS AND IMPLICATIONS

We believe that one of the important contributions of our initial research has been to demonstrate our most basic premise, that among professional women, adult daughter caregivers find their parent-care responsibilities to be both stressful and rewarding. These women do indeed report both types of experiences in their caregiving role. Notably, women more often report rewards from parent care and from other family roles than they report stressors. Findings from our work on women's family roles provide evidence for both the competing demands hypothesis and for the expansion hypothesis. Moreover, our findings underscore the value of considering the quality of role experiences beyond the mere number of family roles occupied to more fully understand the health effects of women's parent-care responsibilities.

Our review of empirical literature on combining parent care and employment strongly suggests that this dual role configuration is not necessarily detrimental to the health of midlife women, as the competing demands hypothesis would suggest. Like many other demanding roles, parent care and employment have the potential to interfere with each other in ways that are harmful to well-being. It is clear, however, that positive experiences in each role, especially in employment, may serve to offset the negative aspects of the other. Most notably, being employed in full-time work that is highly rewarding is likely to buffer the health of adult daughters against the stress of providing care to an ill parent, as the expansion hypothesis would suggest. Thus, this chapter's review of the parent-care and employment literature, including our own contributions, should help allay expressed (and implied) concerns that holding these two roles would be wholly problematic for the well-being of adult daughters (Martire & Stephens, 2003).

Gerontologists have expressed concerns about the effects of parent care and employment on women's well-being and their availability to provide parent care, and employers have expressed concerns about the impact that later life caregiving might have on the midlife workforce and ultimately on productivity. Employees who are providing care to ill family members cost U.S. employers $29 billion annually, which translates into an annual cost of $1,142 per employee. Costs are, in part, a result of decreased productivity, increased turnover rate, and the loss of between 5 and 12 days of work annually. Other sources of these costs stem from the fact that employed caregivers have more stress-related illnesses and use health plans to a greater degree, ultimately adding to costs for the employer in providing health care benefits (U.S. Department of Health and Human Services, Administration on Aging, 2003).

As we have stated previously, the role of history in human development is important. History has had profound effects on the development of multiple roles for women. After we had begun our program of research in the early 1990s, a number of societal and organizational policy developments took place. The U.S. government enacted the Family and Medical

Leave Act of 1993, which assures workers that they can return to jobs after a leave of up to 12 weeks to care for family members with serious health conditions. However, this act guarantees only unpaid leave and generally applies to workers in larger organizations. Other employer benefits that could assist women attempting to balance their parent-care and work roles include flexible work hours, paid sick leave, and vacation days.

Emerging research aimed at evaluating the effects of these legislated and employer-initiated programs reveals some beneficial outcomes for caregivers and employers alike. Women whose employment provides flexible hours, unpaid family leave, and paid sick or vacation days are more likely to remain employed and maintain work hours after assuming the caregiver role than are women whose employers provide fewer benefits (Pavalko & Henderson, 2006). In addition, caregivers are more satisfied with their jobs when their places of employment provide more of these benefits and value the integration of employees' work and family lives (Sahibzada, Hammer, Neal, & Kuang, 2005).

Although employed caregivers who have workplace benefits are likely to remain in the workforce and be satisfied with their work, some research shows that the effects on their well-being stemming from access to these benefits are negligible (Pavalko & Henderson, 2006). Other research shows that female caregivers whose employers offer flexible work arrangements have only marginally better well-being than caregivers without such arrangements (Chesley & Moen, 2006). Even when such employer benefits do not directly affect women's well-being, their effects may be indirect. If such resources allow female caregivers to remain in the labor force and enjoy satisfying work, our research indicates that women's well-being will ultimately be enhanced.

Research, including our own, on employed caregivers has focused most often on women in professional, managerial, or administrative support occupations. We know much less about the effects of juggling parent care and employment for adult daughters who are in occupations that offer less pay, fewer (or no) fringe benefits, little flexibility in work schedules, or few opportunities for career advancement. This issue is important given that caregivers with lower socioeconomic status have poorer well-being (e.g., Meshefedjian, McCusker, Bellavance, & Baumgarten, 1998).

Our review in this chapter has focused separately on the evidence for the competing demands and expansion perspectives, but problematic and positive role experiences are likely to coexist for any given woman. A caregiver is likely to be affected by both the stressful and rewarding aspects of combining her family and work roles. Indeed, our own research, as well as the broader literature on balancing work and family responsibilities, shows that the effects of occupying multiple roles depend heavily on the quality of experiences that transpire within and across these roles. In addition, it can be argued that the accumulation of rewards or demands within and across women's roles affect their well-being throughout their life course (Moen & Chermack, 2005). However, it is likely that the combinations of roles women hold will differ at various life stages, and thus so too will interactions of these roles with their parent-care responsibilities. Moreover, the larger cultural context in which women enact multiple roles also may distinctively affect their well-being (Remennick, 1999).

Findings from our studies provide abundant evidence that the lives of these women cannot be easily captured by either the competing demands or the expansion hypothesis alone. We find the strongest support for competing demands when we focus only on the problems and stressors encountered in the parent-care role and in other family and work roles. Likewise, we find the strongest support for the expansion hypothesis when we focus exclusively on the satisfying and rewarding aspects of role experiences.

A far more complex picture emerges when we consider problematic and rewarding role experiences simultaneously. Our studies have amply demonstrated that positive experiences in one role have the potential to offset the effects of negative experiences in another role. This pattern of findings is not entirely consistent with either the competing demands or with the expansion perspectives.

On the basis of the accumulated findings, we have become convinced that the two questions that guided our original work in this area are more complementary to one another than opposing. Moreover, it is our contention that the processes governing the ways in which multiple roles affect well-being are more complicated than the ones proposed by either role theory. Thus, our research strongly suggests the need for a more comprehensive theoretical framework for understanding the lives of women who are in the middle of parent-care and other roles.

REFERENCES

Ahrens, C. J. C., & Ryff, C. D. (2006). Multiple roles in well-being: Sociodemographic and psychological moderators. *Sex Roles, 55,* 801–815.

Aneshensel, C. S., Pearlin, L. I., Mullan, J. T., Zarit, S. H., & Whitlatch, C. J. (1995). *Profiles in caregiving: The unexpected career.* San Diego, CA: Academic Press.

Atienza, A. A., & Stephens, M. A. P. (2000). Social interactions at work and the well-being of daughters involved in parent care. *Journal of Applied Gerontology, 19,* 243–263.

Barnett, R., & Baruch, G. (1985). Women's involvement in multiple roles and psychological distress. *Journal of Personality and Social Psychology, 49,* 135–145.

Barnett, R. C., & Marshall, N. L. (1992). Worker and mother roles, spillover effects and psychological distress. *Women and Health, 18,* 9–40.

Boyd, S. L., & Treas, J. (1989). Family care of the frail elderly: A new look at "women in the middle." *Women's Studies Quarterly, 1–2,* 66–74.

Brody, E. M. (1981). "Women in the middle" and family help to older people. *The Gerontologist, 21,* 471–480.

Brody, E. M. (1985). Parent care as a normative family stress. *The Gerontologist, 25,* 19–29.

Brody, E. M. (1990). *Women in the middle: Their parent-care years.* New York: Springer Publishing Company.

Brody, E. M. (2004). *Women in the middle: Their parent care years* (2nd ed.). New York: Springer Publishing Company.

Chesley, N., & Moen, P. (2006). When workers care: Dual-earner couples' caregiving strategies, benefit use, and psychological well-being. *American Behavioral Scientist, 49,* 1248–1269.

Enright, R. B., & Friss, L. (1987). *Employed caregivers of brain-impaired adults.* San Francisco: Family Survival Project.

Etaugh, C. A., & Bridges, J. S. (2006). Midlife transitions. In J. Worell & C. D. Goodheart (Eds.), *Handbook of girls' and women's psychological health* (pp. 359–367). New York: Oxford University Press.

The Family and Medical Leave Act of 1993, Public Law 103-3, 29 U.S.C., ch. 28, enacted February 5, 1993.

Franks, M. M., & Stephens, M. A. P. (1992). Multiple roles of middle generation caregivers: Contextual effects and psychological mechanisms. *Journal of Gerontology: Social Sciences, 47,* 123–129.

Franks, M. M., & Stephens, M. A. P. (1996). Social support in the context of caregiving: Husbands' provision of support to wives involved in parent care. *Journals of Gerontology: Psychological Sciences, 51B,* 43–52.

Giele, J. Z., Mutschler, P. H., & Orodenker, S. Z. (1987). *Stress and burdens of caregiving for the frail elderly* (Working Paper No. 36). Waltham, MA: Brandeis University.

Gignac, M. A. M., Kelloway, E. K., & Gottlieb, B. H. (1996). The impact of caregiving on employment: A mediational model of work–family conflict. *Canadian Journal on Aging, 15,* 525–542.

Goode, W. J. (1960). A theory of role strain. *American Sociological Review, 25,* 483–496.

He, W., Sengupta, M., Velkoff, V. A., & DeBarros, K. A. (2005). *65+ in the United States: 2005.* Retrieved June 7, 2006, from http://www.census.gov/prod/2006pubs/p23-209.pdf

Marks, S. R. (1977). Multiple roles and role strain: Some notes on human energy, time and commitment. *American Sociological Review, 42,* 921–936.

Martire, L. M., & Stephens, M. A. P. (2003). Juggling parent care and employment responsibilities: The dilemmas of adult daughter caregivers in the work force. *Sex Roles: A Journal of Research, 48,* 167–173.

Martire, L. M., Stephens, M. A. P., & Atienza, A. A. (1997). The interplay of work and caregiving: Relationships between role satisfaction, role involvement, and caregivers' well-being. *Journal of Gerontology: Social Sciences, 52B,* S279–S289.

Martire, L. M., Stephens, M. A. P., & Townsend, A. L. (2000). Centrality of women's multiple roles: Beneficial and detrimental consequences for psychological well-being. *Psychology and Aging, 15,* 148–156.

Meshefedjian, G., McCusker, J., Bellavance, F., & Baumgarten, M. (1998). Factors associated with symptoms of depression among informal caregivers of demented elders in the community. *The Gerontologist, 38,* 247–253.

MetLife Mature Market Institute, National Alliance for Caregiving, & The National Center on Women and Aging. (1999, November). *The Metlife Juggling Act Study: Balancing caregiving with work and the costs involved.* Retrieved June 28, 2006, from http://www.metlife.com/WPSAssets/12949500261100547900V1FJuggling%20Study%20-111004.pdf

Miller, B. (1989). Adult children's perceptions of caregiver stress and satisfaction. *Journal of Applied Gerontology, 8,* 275–293.

Mitchell, V., & Helson, R. (1990). Women's prime of life: Is it the 50s? *Psychology of Women Quarterly, 14,* 451–470.

Moen, P., & Chermack, K. (2005). Gender disparities in health: Strategic selection, careers, and cycles of control. *Journal of Gerontology: Social Sciences, 60B,* 99–108.

Moen, P., Robinson, J., & Fields, V. (1994). Women's work and caregiving roles: A life course approach. *Journal of Gerontology, 49*, 176–186.

Neal, M. B., Chapman, N. J., Ingersoll-Dayton, B., & Emlen, A. C. (1993*). Balancing work and caregiving for children, adults, and elders.* Newbury Park, CA: Sage.

Norton, T. R., Gupta, A., Stephens, M. A. P., Martire, L. M., & Townsend A. L. (2005). Stress, rewards, and change in the centrality of women's family and work roles: Mastery as a mediator. *Sex Roles, 52*, 325–335.

Norton, T. R., Stephens, M. A. P., Martire, L. M., Townsend, A. L., & Gupta, A. (2002). Change in the centrality of women's' multiple roles: Effects of role stress and rewards. *Journal of Gerontology: Social Sciences, 57B*, S52–S62.

Pavalko, E. K., & Henderson, K. A. (2006). Combining care work and paid work: Do workplace policies make a difference? *Research on Aging, 28*, 359–374.

Pavalko, E. K., & Woodbury, S. (2000). Social roles as process: Caregiving careers and women's health. *Journal of Health and Social Behavior, 41*, 91–105.

Remennick, L. I. (1999). Women of the "sandwich" generation and multiple roles: The case of Russian immigrants of the 1990s in Israel. *Sex Roles, 40*, 347–378.

Rosenthal, C. J., Matthews, S. H., & Marshall, V. W. (1989). Is parent care normative? The experiences of a sample of middle-aged women. *Research on Aging, 11*, 224–260.

Ross, C. E., & Mirowsky, M. (1995). Does employment affect health? *Journal of Health and Social Behavior, 36*, 230–243.

Sahibzada, K., Hammer, L. B., Neal, M. B., & Kuang, D. C. (2005). The moderating effects of work–family role combinations and work–family organizational culture on the relationship between family-friendly workplace supports and job satisfaction. *Journal of Family Issues, 26*, 820–839.

Skaff, M. M., & Pearlin, L. I. (1992). Caregiving: Role engulfment and the loss of self. *The Gerontologist, 32*, 656–664.

Spitze, G., & Logan, J. (1990). More evidence on women (and men) in the middle. *Research on Aging, 12*, 182–198.

Stephens, M. A. P., & Franks, M. M. (1995). Spillover between daughters' roles as caregiver and wife: Interference or enhancement? *Journal of Gerontology: Psychological Sciences, 50B*, 9–17.

Stephens, M. A. P., Franks, M. M., & Atienza, A. A. (1997). Where two roles intersect: Spillover between parent care and employment. *Psychology and Aging, 12*, 30–37.

Stephens, M. A. P., Franks, M. M., & Townsend, A. L. (1994). Stress and rewards in women's multiple roles: The case of women in the middle. *Psychology and Aging, 9*, 45–52.

Stephens, M. A. P., & Townsend, A. L. (1997). Stress of parent care: Positive and negative effects of women's other roles. *Psychology and Aging, 12*, 376–386.

Stephens, M. A. P., Townsend, A. L., Martire, L. M., & Druley, J. A. (2001). Balancing parent care with other roles: Interrole conflict of adult daughter caregivers. *Journal of Gerontology: Psychological Sciences, 56B,* P24–P34.

Stoller, E. P., & Pugliesi, K. L. (1989). The transition to the caregiving role. *Research on Aging, 11,* 312–330.

Thoits, P. A. (1992). Identity structures and psychological well-being: Gender and marital status comparisons. *Social Psychology Quarterly, 55,* 236–256.

U.S. Bureau of the Census. (2006, September 21). *America's families and living arrangements: 2005.* Retrieved June 23, 2006, from http://www.census.gov/population/www/socdemo/hh-fam/cps2005.html

U.S. Department of Health and Human Services, Administration on Aging. (2003, August 27). *National Family Caregiver Support Program.* Retrieved June 7, 2006, from http://www.aoa.gov/press/fact/pdf/ss_nfcsp.pdf

Waldron, I., & Jacobs, J. A. (1989). Effects of multiple roles on women's health: Evidence from a national longitudinal study. *Women and Health, 15,* 3–19.

Wethington, E., & Kessler, R. C. (1989). Employment, parental responsibility, and psychological distress: A longitudinal study of married women. *Journal of Family Issues, 10,* 527–546.

Wolff, J. L., & Kasper, J. D. (2006). Caregivers of frail elders: Updating a national profile. *The Gerontologist, 46,* 344–356.

6

The Importance of Context and the Gain–Loss Dynamic for Understanding Grandparent Caregivers

Julie Hicks Patrick and Eric A. Goedereis

The role of grandparenting in the United States historically has not been clearly defined. Early research addressed various styles of grandparenting (Cherlin & Furstenberg, 1986; Neugarten & Weinstein, 1964), noting that grandparents often served as a "family watchdog," observing from the sidelines and ready to step in when needed (Troll, 1985). In recent decades, many Americans have found it necessary to return to active parenting, living with and helping to raise their young grandchildren. In the current chapter, we discuss the challenges and rewards these grandparent caregivers face. In keeping with the theme of this volume, we view these concerns from the "lens of life span development" (Hayslip & Patrick, 2003).

Life span development involves many principles, chief of which are the ideas that development is a life-long process, marked by both gains and losses; that development is influenced by the historical and cultural context in which it occurs; and that development occurs along multiple dimensions and is influenced by multiple factors (Baltes, 1987, 1997). Thus, as Hayslip and Patrick (2003) have argued, the life span development framework may be the most appropriate one in which to examine the varying antecedents and multidimensional consequences grandparent caregivers experience. Several aspects of the life span framework are particularly salient for understanding the experiences of the members of this group, including the role of history and context, increased hetero-geneity via nonnormative life events and individual difference factors, and the importance of mutual and reciprocal influences (Baltes, 1987; Lerner, 1996; Riegel, 1976).

DEFINING GRANDPARENT CAREGIVING

The U.S. Census Bureau has estimated that of the 56 million Americans who are grandparents, 5.7 million live with their young grandchildren. In more than 40% (2.4 million) of these coresident dyads, the grandparent has primary responsibility for the grandchild's basic needs. Census data also indicate that among grandparent-headed households, 50% include both grandparents, about 43% include a grandmother only, and approxi-mately 6% include a grandfather only (U.S. Census Bureau, 2005).

Although there is no established nomenclature for describing the diversity among grandparent-headed households, many researchers have classified grandparent caregivers along a continuum that incorporates the type and frequency of care provided as well as the legal status of the caregivers. One particularly useful classification is that of Fuller-Thomson and Minkler (2000). Using the National Survey of Families and Households data set, they determined that of American grandparents, 40.4% are noncaregivers. Another 47.5% can be termed intermediate caregivers, providing up to 29 hours of care per week. These families include both three-generation households and "skip generation" fami-lies, in which the parents are not coresident. An additional 6.8% of the grandparents provide full care for a grandchild in the absence of a legal custody arrangement, and 5.3% have sole legal custody of their grand-children (Fuller-Thomson & Minkler, 2000). A similar classification, based on current coresidence, current versus previous primary responsi-bility, and the level of care provided, has been suggested by R. D. Lee, Ensminger, and LaVeist (2006) to describe grandparent caregiving more accurately. Using this fine-grained classification, more than two thirds of the grandmothers were providing moderate to high levels of child care to grandchildren.

HISTORICAL AND SOCIAL CONTEXT

Multigenerational residences are not unique to our current historical period, although the structure and reasons for coresidence may be influenced by our current social and economic milieu (R. D. Lee et al., 2006). For example, in previous cohorts, young married couples might have moved into the residence of a parent during the early years of their marriage or in times of economic hardship. Once the young couple began to establish themselves financially, they would move into their own residence. In 1970, families with two parents and children represented about 40% of American households. By 2000, this structure characterized only 24% of American households (Fields & Casper, 2001). The nation experienced a 118% increase in grandparent–grandchild coresidence during the same period (Casper & Bryson, 1998; Szinovacz, 1998). In many of these families, grandparents share child-rearing responsibilities with a parent; in approximately 40% of these families, grandparents have sole responsibility for the grandchild (Casper & Bryson, 1998).

Grandparents assume a major caregiving role for a number of reasons that are unique to the current cohort. The dramatic increase from previous cohorts is the result of increased substance abuse in the parent generation, incarceration among parents (especially mothers), HIV/AIDS, single-parent households, long work hours and job demands of the middle generation, high rates of childbirth among adolescents, military service, and legal preference for kinship care over foster care (Backhouse, 2006; McGowen, Ladd, & Strom, 2006).

In contrast to providing care for an aging parent who has experienced an acute or disabling medical event, simultaneous crises often precipitate entry into grandparent caregiving. For many grandparents, assuming the caregiving role was a gradual process influenced by multiple factors. For example, in one qualitative study of grandmother caregivers, 31% of the coresident grandmothers and 24% of nonresident grandmothers reported that substance abuse was the major factor leading to the assumption of the caregiver role. In addition, 50% of the coresident and 52% of the nonresident grandmothers cited the middle generation's employment situation as an important factor. A majority (57%) of the coresident grandmothers also listed domestic violence as a reason for assuming care (McGowen et al., 2006).

UNIQUE CONCERNS
OF GRANDPARENT CAREGIVERS

In addition to stressors that are common across caregiving contexts, grandparent caregivers face unique challenges. Specifically, they often report feeling "off-time" from their age peers who are no longer involved in daily child care as well as feeling off-time from the parents of the grandchild's classmates who are significantly younger and engaging in age normative child care (Backhouse, 2006; Minkler, Fuller-Thomson, Miller, & Driver, 1997). This is an especially intriguing yet unexplored area. Baird (2003) wrote eloquently in her dual role of grandparent caregiver and scholar about the anger, exhaustion, and disappointment that she felt when she took on this role and that continued to color her experiences raising her grandchild. She described the feeling that same-aged peers may view the role of grandparent caregiving as "their worst nightmare" (Baird, 2003, p. 61).

Similar to the stigma experienced by parents and other caregivers to adults with schizophrenia and other chronic mental illnesses (Patrick & Hayden, 1999), grandparent caregivers must cope with their own and others' (Baird, 2003) doubts and opinions about the effectiveness of their own parenting. Many deal with a wealth of unsolicited advice from others. This notable lack of support from others is an important but understudied area among grandparent caregivers.

To understand the kinds of suggestions offered to caregiving grandparents facing high child care demands, Strough, Patrick, and Swenson (2003) presented two hypothetical grandparenting vignettes to 112 adults. One vignette featured a grandmother who was often asked to babysit for three young grandchildren and was beginning to feel that her adult child was taking advantage of her. The second vignette featured a couple who were increasingly concerned about their daughter's substance abuse and the possibility that their grandchild was being neglected. In both cases, participants were asked to state what the grandparent should do. In the babysitting

CONTEXT AND THE GAIN–LOSS DYNAMIC

vignette, significant differences did not emerge in the number or type of problem-solving strategies offered by those with and without previous experience in these situations. For such common and mild grandparenting problems, most people agreed that the grandmother needed to assert her position and suggest alternate child-care arrangements to the parents. However, in the case of the grandparents who were concerned about the substance abuse and neglectful parenting of their adult daughter, previous experience was an important factor related to the type of problem-solving strategies that were offered. Those with prior experience were more likely to suggest seeking outside assistance and less likely to suggest trying to change the daughter's behavior than were those without such personal experience. Strough et al. interpreted these findings to suggest that it matters from whom grandparents receive advice and support.

Another unique aspect of grandparent caregiving is the expressed frustration related to different norms for child behavior and parenting across generations (Backhouse, 2006; Baird, 2003; Bullock, 2005; Patrick & Tomczewski, 2007; Strom & Strom, 2000). Although well socialized into the role of parent, few grandparents enter the role of caregiver with current information about communication skills, sexually transmitted diseases, attention-deficit/hyperactivity disorder, behavioral problems, or effective ways to help children deal with grief and anger (Hayslip, 2003; Roberto & Qualls, 2003). Evidence suggests that parent training for grandparent caregivers can provide needed assistance to the grandparents (Hayslip, 2003; Kern, 2003). Indeed, among members of grandparent support groups, many value the opportunity to refresh and retool their parenting skills (Smith, 2003). However, just as caregivers of older adults face barriers to attending support groups, so do grandparent caregivers (Roberto & Qualls).

Grandparent caregivers also face a high level of social and legal ambiguity related to the permanence of their custodial relationship with their grandchild, with an omnipresent concern that the parents or others may nullify or compromise the caregiving arrangement (Baird, 2003; Generations United, 2000; Karp, 1996; Smith, 2003).

The grandchildren themselves pose unique caregiving challenges. A majority (73%) of the grandchildren raised by grandparents are less than 6 years old (Casper & Bryson, 1998; Fuller-Thomson & Minkler,

2000); boys are overrepresented (Hayslip, Shore, & Lambert, 1998). In an examination of African American grandmothers participating in the National Survey of Families and Households study, Fuller-Thomson and Minkler (2000) reported that more than half of the grandmothers (54%) began primary care of their grandchild before the child's 1st birthday. Another 20% began care when the grandchild was between 1 and 5 years of age, and 17% began when the grandchild was 5 to 10 years of age. An additional 8% entered the caregiver role when the grandchild was age 11 years or older. The influence of these contextual factors on the grandparent caregiver and the grandchild whom they are raising cannot be overestimated. Different stages of child development and varying circumstances exert profound effects on the grandparent and grandchild as they negotiate new relationships with each other and with other family members.

To further complicate the caregiving context, about half of all grandparent caregivers are raising more than one grandchild (Joslin & Brouard, 1995; Minkler & Roe, 1993). Because researchers typically ask grandparent caregivers to focus on one grandchild for research purposes (Hayslip & Patrick, 2003), little is known about the families in which grandparent caregivers are raising multiple grandchildren.

WELL-BEING AMONG GRANDPARENT CAREGIVERS

Higher psychological well-being is typically characterized by high levels of positive emotions and experiences, high life satisfaction, and infrequent negative emotions and experiences (Diener, Suh, Lucas, & Smith, 1999). Determination of physical well-being typically includes global assessments of health, physical activities, and specific numbers and types of chronic health conditions. Across caregiving contexts, family caregivers are at risk for negative psychological and health effects. As is often found in the broader caregiving literature, grandparent caregivers often assume the role to the detriment of their own physical and psychological well-being (Hayslip, Shore, & Emick, 2006; Strawbridge, Wallhagen, Shema, & Kaplan, 1997).

DIFFERENCES BETWEEN
CAREGIVER GRANDPARENTS
AND NONCAREGIVER GRANDPARENTS

Given the likelihood of coresidence and the child-care responsibilities associated with the role, caregiving grandparents differ from noncaregiving grandparents along a number of dimensions. First and foremost are differences in role satisfaction and role meaning. Hayslip et al. (1998) compared groups of grandparents and found that men in all groups reported more positive grandparenting experiences, whereas among women, noncaregiving grandmothers had the highest satisfaction scores. McGowen et al. (2006) also found that caregiving grandparents reported less satisfaction with grandparenting and a lower sense of being successful than noncaregiving grandparents who coresided with young grandchildren. Many grandparent caregivers reported feeling cheated of the traditional grandparenting role that they had envisioned for themselves (Baird, 2003; Smith, 2003).

Grandparent caregivers often assume the role at significant personal cost to their own well-being. Relative to noncaregiving grandparents, grandparent caregivers report more symptoms of depression (Fuller-Thomson & Minkler, 2000; Minkler et al., 1997; Musil, 1998). Grandmothers who are the primary caregivers reported experiencing significantly more parenting stress than those with only part-time responsibility (Musil, 1998). Full-time grandmother caregivers also reported seeking less social support than part-time grandmother caregivers (Musil, 1998; Young & Dawson, 2003).

Relative to noncaregiving age peers, caregiving grandmothers have been found to have worse physical health (Fuller-Thomson & Minkler, 2000; Hayslip et al., 1998; Solomon & Marx, 1998). S. Lee, Colditz, Berkman, & Kawachi (2003), using data from the Nurses Health Study, found that the negative health effects accruing to grandmother caregivers have been observed among women providing even low to moderate levels of care. Grandmothers providing 9 or more hours per week of care to a non-ill grandchild were 1.5 times more likely to have heart disease compared with those who were not assisting grandchildren.

In terms of external resources to support them, caregiving grandparents are more likely to have low educational attainment, be employed, work longer hours, and have less total household income than homes without grandchildren present (U.S. Census Bureau, 2005; Wang & Marcotte, 2007). Thus, grandparent caregivers experience a host of negative social, psychological, and health effects.

Although comparisons between grandparent caregivers and other family caregivers are rare, Strawbridge et al. (1997) provided an exception. They compared the physical and psychological well-being of 42 grandparent caregivers, 44 spouse caregivers, and 130 adult child caregivers with more than 1,600 noncaregivers over a 20-year period. All three groups of caregivers exhibited poorer psychological well-being relative to noncaregivers. When compared with spouse and adult child caregivers, grandparent caregivers also experienced poorer physical health and had experienced more negative life events than their caregiving peers.

EXPLAINING AND PREDICTING WELL-BEING AMONG GRANDPARENT CAREGIVERS

Most studies examining the experiences of grandparent caregivers have relied on a stress and coping model, although a few studies have used other frameworks (e.g., Carr, 2006; Patrick & Pickard, 2003; Pruchno & McKenney, 2006). All of these approaches can be situated within the life span development framework. At its most basic level, the stress and coping framework (Lazarus & Folkman, 1984) includes an explicit examination of background characteristics and resources, stressors, moderators such as social support and formal support, attributions and perceptions, and physical and psychological well-being outcomes. Indeed, this general model has guided much of the family caregiving literature over the past 3 decades.

The stress and coping framework is modified somewhat when applied to the experiences of grandparent caregivers, although its use is similar to that of other groups of family caregivers. Level of care, on a continuum from babysitting to full-time custodial care, is often included as a design feature guiding participant recruitment (R. D. Lee et al., 2006). Because of the nature of grandparenting, the age range of grandparent caregivers is often larger than that found in studies of spouse or adult child caregivers (Goodman, 2006). Grandparent caregiving research typically expands the range of stressors to include behavioral problems, cognitive challenges, medical issues, and emotional problems exhibited by the young grandchild (Crowther & Rodriguez, 2003; Emick & Hayslip, 1996; Kinney, McGrew, & Nelson, 2003; Kolomer, 2000).

INDIVIDUAL DIFFERENCES AMONG GRANDPARENT CAREGIVERS

Although it is rare to directly compare grandparent outcomes as a function of the reasons for assuming the role, the limited evidence available suggests that these reasons affect the levels of stressors experienced. For example, grandparents who were giving care as a result of their children's substance abuse, incarceration, or AIDS status received less social support and had poorer outcomes than grandparents who assumed the role because of their children's marital and financial disruptions (Musil, 1998; Young & Dawson, 2003). Among caregiving grandmothers, those raising grandchildren with no behavior problems had higher scores than those whose coresident grandchildren presented behavior problems (Hayslip et al., 1998). Outcomes were worse in low-income families, when no spouse was available and when other young children resided in the same house.

More is known about the ways in which individual characteristics of the grandparent caregivers operate within the stress and coping model. Therefore, we selectively review the state of the art in terms of four individual difference factors: age, race, gender, and education.

Age

In census reports, grandparent caregivers have ranged in age from 30 years to more than 90 years (Simmons & Dye, 2003). Some 28% were aged 60 and older, but most were between the ages of 50 and 59 years (Simmons & Dye, 2003). It is precisely this stage of middle age during which health concerns become especially prominent (Brim, Ryff, & Kessler, 2004).

Whether their physical health will allow them to continue providing care to grandchildren has been a frequently cited concern of grandparent caregivers (Baird, 2003; Bullock, 2005; McCallion & Kolomer, 2006; McGowen et al., 2006; Smith, 2003). Thus, in terms of physical and psychological functioning, age may exert both direct and indirect effects on the well-being of grandparent caregivers.

Consistent with models related to the life span approach, the association between age and well-being among grandparent caregivers is more complex than a simple negative linear relationship. For example, Goodman (2006) examined the influence of age in a sample of more than 1,000 grandmothers in the Los Angeles area. About half of the grandmothers, who ranged in age from 37 years to 86 years, were primary caregivers, and the remaining were coparenting with their sons and daughters. Analyses revealed that those grandmothers older than 65 years seemed to be faring better than their middle-aged and younger counterparts, especially when losses related to physical aging were statistically controlled. Consistent with socioemotional selectivity theory (Carstensen, Isaacowitz, & Charles, 1999), the older grandmothers reported less distress related to dysfunction in their own children and less distress related to problem behaviors exhibited by their grandchildren (Goodman, 2006).

Race

The literature on grandparent caregivers is replete with the statement that the phenomenon of raising one's grandchildren cuts across racial and economic lines. Although true, the statement is somewhat misleading. In the 2000 U.S. census, the first to explicitly include questions on grandparent caregivers, only 2% of non-Hispanic White adults reported living with a grandchild; 42% reported having primary responsibility for the coresident grandchild. In contrast, 6% of Asian adults, 8% of Native American and Alaskan Native adults, 8% of Black adults, 8% of Hispanic adults, and 10% of Pacific Islander adults reported living with a grandchild (Simmons & Dye, 2003). Although coresident, Hispanic adults (35%) were less likely than Blacks (52%) or Native American/Alaskan Natives (56%) to be caregivers. On the basis of data from more than 3,200 grandparent-headed households in the Panel Study of Income Dynamics, Wang and Marcotte (2007) found that Blacks were 1.8 times more likely to be grandparent caregivers than were Whites. In terms of geographic distribution, approximately 48% of grandparent caregivers reside in the South (Simmons & Dye, 2003).

When race differences in well-being outcomes have emerged among grandparent caregivers, the direction has been equivocal. Currently, there is research showing no race differences in well-being (Goldberg-Glen & Sands, 2000), more stress among White grandmothers (Pruchno, 1999), and particularly high levels of depressive symptoms among Black grandmothers (Fuller-Thomson & Minkler, 2000). One reason for such mixed results likely rests with the importance of normative and nonnormative life events. For many women, including Hispanic grandmothers (Goodman, 2006; Hayslip, Baird, Toledo, Toledo, & Emick, 2006) and Black grandmothers (Kohn & Smith, 2006), the role of grandmother caregiver is neither negative nor unexpected. Many report having been raised by their own grandparents and view this extended family arrangement as ideal (Crowther & Rodriguez, 2003).

Gender

Early research on grandparenting showed that men and women view the role differently and derive different levels and sources of satisfaction, with men reporting higher levels of satisfaction with grandparenting than women (Thomas, 1989). These differences, however, are often associated with differences in role expectations (Hayslip, Temple, Shore, & Henderson, 2006). Given that at least 64% of grandparent caregivers are women (Simmons & Dye, 2003), gender is an important individual difference variable to examine among grandparent caregivers.

Among grandfathers with primary responsibility for a grandchild's basic needs, 41% are age 60 and older, approximately 71% are married, and more than 70% are employed (U.S. Census Bureau, 2005). Although the economic plight of caregiving grandmothers is well known, grandfather caregivers face similar challenges. Men in grandfather-only households are less likely to be employed, less likely to own their homes, more likely to be

Black, and more likely to be poor compared with married grandfather caregivers (U.S. Census Bureau, 2005; Patrick & Tomczewski, 2007).

In recent studies contrasting the psychological well-being of grandparent caregivers, grandfathers reported more depressive symptoms and lower levels of social support than grandmothers (Hayslip, Kaminski, & Earnheart, 2006). They also reported more disruptions in their lives because of child care than grandmother caregivers (Szinovacz & Davey, 2006). Like grandmother caregivers, caregiving grandfathers found both uplifts and challenges in the role. Most grandfathers expressed a desire to be an active part of their coresident grandchild's life and a sense of generativity, in that they valued the life lessons that they could teach their young grandchildren. However, caregiving grandfathers may also experience a loss of freedom as a result of child-care responsibilities (McCallion & Kolomer, 2006), feel challenged by differences in current child-care practices from their own days as parents, and feel fearful regarding future health declines (Bullock, 2005). Many caregiving grandfathers also have reported feeling powerless in their role, a result not reported in the literature on grandmothers (Bullock, 2005).

Education and Employment

The current cohort of middle-aged and older adults has experienced marked changes in educational and occupational opportunities compared with previous generations, and this is especially evident for women. These women are among the first to struggle with the demands of balancing work and family (Carr, 2004).

Although grandparent caregivers are more likely to be employed than noncaregiving age peers (Wang & Marcotte, 2007), this trend is moderated by grandparent gender. Among all grandparents, a decrease in the number of hours worked tends to occur as the person neared retirement. For married grandfather caregivers, this decrease in hours worked is slower because men are more likely to postpone retirement. For grandmother caregivers, the drop is much steeper (Wang & Marcotte, 2007). This trend is clarified by Pruchno and McKenney's (2006) findings that caregiving grandmothers face and resolve work disruptions in a number of ways. In that study, many women simply exited the workforce as a means to resolve work and family demands. Those women who remained employed reported both more time away from work and working longer hours. It is interesting that women with more years of education reported more work disruptions; whether this seeming contradiction is a function of the women trying to "make up" for time away from the job or is a function of the kinds of jobs the women hold remains an empirical question to be examined. The finding is particularly intriguing in light of other research showing that grandmother caregivers with lower levels of educational attainment report higher satisfaction in the role (Hayslip et al., 1998). Future studies may help clarify whether this counterintuitive result is cohort specific. Such trends may be unique to this current cohort of grandmother caregivers, who were among the first to experience such high family demands and expanding employment opportunities.

EFFECTS ON GRANDCHILDREN

A true life span perspective on grandparent caregivers would acknowledge that caregiving occurs within a rich and multidimensional context by including more of the people involved with the grandparent caregiver, such as the grandchild being raised, middle-generation parents, and non-resident grandchildren and their parents. To date, little information about the effects on these important family members is available.

In terms of grandchild outcomes, most service providers, clinicians, and researchers recognize that many grandchildren who are being raised by grandparents have experienced stressful life events. For some children, these stressful environments begin during gestation. Thus, grandchildren being raised by grandparents may enter the caregiving relationship with significant impediments to their emotional and physical well-being (Mackintosh, Myers, & Kennon, 2006). Because the challenges are so varied and because problem behaviors may be idiosyncratic, it is difficult to identify an appropriate comparison group by which to assess the effects of grandparent caregiving on the children. Although high-quality data on grandchild outcomes are scarce, results of a meta-analysis suggest that there are no harmful effects on children reared in kinship care arrangements (Winokur, Rozen, Thompson, Green, & Valentine, 2005). In fact, these children fare better than those in foster care on a range of indices, including behavior problems, reentry to the social service system, adaptive behaviors, family relations, and mental health (Winokur et al., 2005). In a small study with a clinical sample of families seeking substance abuse treatment for their coresident adolescents, grandparent caregivers reported fewer problems with delinquency, lower monitoring of teen behavior, and fewer interpersonal conflicts than did mothers (Robbins, Briones, Schwartz, Dillon, & Mitrani, 2006).

The effects of being raised by a grandparent are likely to extend beyond the period of coresidence. A new question being posed in the literature is whether those raised by their grandparents will be more likely to assume kin care in their own futures. We are beginning to tackle this issue in our own lab, examining emerging adults' attitudes and perceptions toward grandparent caregiving. Specifically, we are examining whether early coresidence with a grandparent and the extent of child rearing by grandparents influence the acceptability of grandparent caregiving. Patrick, Hayslip, and Tomczewski (2008) recently collected data from 269 emerging adults enrolled in a psychology course at a large mid-Atlantic university. The sample included 93 men and 176 women with a mean age of 19.98 years ($SD = 1.78$; range = 18 to 33 years). Typical of the region, 91.2% of the participants were White. Participants responded to an online survey that asked for general background information such as age and gender and contained a series of yes–no items relating to whether they lived at a grandparent's home when younger, whether a grandparent lived with their family when younger, and whether the grandparent helped to raise them. Participants also read a brief vignette and answered 75 closed-ended follow-up questions about the vignette using a 5-point Likert-type scale (1= *strongly disagree*, 5 = *strongly agree*). One area of interest germane to the purposes of this chapter was whether these emerging adults would favor grandparent–grandchild coresidence for themselves if they were the middle-generation parent, whether they would favor this arrangement if they were the grandparent, and whether they would prefer a three-generation arrangement if they were the grandparent.

On the basis of census estimates of coresidence with grandparents (U.S. Census Bureau, 2005), it was expected that approximately 10% of the sample would report having been coresident with a grandparent. In the sample of emerging adults, however, 22.3% indicated that a grandparent had lived with their family when they were younger, and 20.1% indicated that they had lived at a grandparent's house when younger. Furthermore, a cross-tabulation showed that a total of 84 adults (31.2%) had been coresident with a grandparent at some time. When asked whether a grandparent had helped to raise them, 39.8% responded affirmatively. Thus, the sample was divided into four groups: traditional families (i.e., nonresident and low child care; 46.1%), nonresident but high child care (22.7%), coresident but low child care (14.1%), and coresident and high child care (17.1%).

In terms of their overall comfort with grandparent caregiving in their own lives, it had been expected that previous coresidence with a grandparent would be associated with stronger endorsements. However, few significant differences emerged. With regard to their comfort with coresidence if they were the grandparent, the sample mean was moderate ($M = 3.26$, $SD = 1.16$) overall. Results of a one-way analysis of variance showed a significant overall effect of previous experience, $F(3, 265) = 4.01$, $p < .01$. Post hoc tests revealed that those experiencing coresident–high child care grandparents were significantly more likely than those experiencing traditional grandparents to report feeling comfortable becoming grandparent caregivers themselves. No other group differences emerged. Mean endorsement of feeling comfortable with coresidence as the middle generation parent was moderate ($M = 2.98$, $SD = 1.26$). Comfort with multigenerational living arrangements was also moderate ($M = 3.02$, $SD = 1.32$).

Although these results are preliminary, they offer promise for understanding the ways in which grandchildren experience long-lasting effects as a result of living with and being raised by grandparents. Additional analyses may help clarify the mechanism through which Black and Hispanic grandparents, who often experience grandparenting as a normative event, deal effectively with the demands of living with and helping to raise young grandchildren. Finally, the results also are a reminder that a goal for most grandparent caregivers is to minimize differences between their custodial charges and children raised by their own parents.

SUMMARY

The principles of life span development emphasize that multiple gains and losses occur simultaneously across all periods of development (Baltes, 1987). The net balance of these gains and losses is determined, in part, by the context in which one lives. Key contextual factors that increase heterogeneity among adults include normative age-graded events, sociocultural influences, and nonnormative life events (Baltes, 1987). With these aspects in mind, the life span approach may be particularly useful for understanding the challenges and rewards experienced by grandparent caregivers (Hayslip & Patrick, 2003).

Age, gender, race, and education are among the contextual factors that relate to the physical and psychological well-being of grandparent caregivers. As life span theory would predict, the associations are complex. For example, grandparent caregivers experience poorer physical health than noncaregiving grandparents (R. D. Lee et al., 2006). Many would assume that advanced age exacerbates this association. However, as Goodman's (2006) data demonstrate, younger and middle-aged grandparent caregivers fare more poorly than their older counterparts. Possible explanations for this result may be found in *socioemotional selectivity theory* (Carstensen et al., 1999), which posits that with increased age, fewer social demands free up energy for people's most cherished relationships. This pruning of the social network is also accompanied by a more temperate emotional experience. Thus, in light of this theory, it is not surprising that the oldest grandmother caregivers reported fewer interpersonal problems with their coresident adolescent grandchildren (Goodman, 2006).

The tenets of life span development also take into account the increased heterogeneity among adults. This is borne out in the grandparent caregiver literature by contrasting the experiences of women who view the role of grandparent caregiver as a nonnormative life event with those who view it as a continuation of existing family patterns. For example, Hayslip et al. (2006) and Goodman (2006) noted that among Hispanic women and Black women, respectively, grandparent caregiving is not viewed as a disruptive life event. Acknowledging such differences within and across groups of grandparent caregivers may significantly advance our understanding of vulnerability and the variations in grandparent outcomes.

Although the research on grandparent caregivers has expanded to include large and diverse samples and to use sophisticated analyses, the principles of life span development need to be applied more fully in research. We encourage researchers to make use of newer analytic tools, including those for dyadic data and nested models, to examine more fully how the grandparent caregiver relationship affects other family members. These tools used with a dialectical approach may begin to elicit a true understanding of the ways context and the gain–loss dynamic affects grandparent caregivers.

REFERENCES

Backhouse, J. (2006, October). *Grandparents as parents: Social change and its impact on grandparents who are raising their grandchildren.* Paper presented at the Social Change in the 21st Century Conference, Queensland University of Technology, Queensland, Australia.

Baird, A. H. (2003). Through my eyes: Service needs of grandparents who raise their grandchildren, from the perspective of a custodial grandmother. In B. Hayslip, Jr., & J. H. Patrick (Eds.), *Working with custodial grandparents* (pp. 59–65). New York: Springer Publishing Company.

Baltes, P. B. (1987). Theoretical propositions of life span developmental psychology: On the dynamics of growth and decline. *Developmental Psychology, 23,* 611–626.

Baltes, P. B. (1997). On the incomplete architecture of human ontogeny: Selection, optimization and compensation as foundation of developmental theory. *American Psychologist, 52,* 366–380.

Brim, O. G., Ryff, C. D., & Kessler, R. C. (Eds.). (2004). *How healthy are we? A national study of well-being at midlife.* Chicago: University of Chicago Press.

Bullock, K. (2005). Grandfathers and the impact of raising grandchildren. *Journal of Sociology & Social Welfare, 32,* 43–59.

Carr, D. (2004). Psychological well-being across three cohorts: A response to shifting work–family opportunities and expectations? In O. G. Brim, C. D. Ryff & R. C. Kessler (Eds.), *How healthy are we? A national study of well-being at midlife* (pp. 452–484). Chicago: University of Chicago Press.

Carr, G. F. (2006). Vulnerability: A conceptual model of African American grand-mother caregivers. *Journal of Theory Construction and Testing, 10,* 11–14.

Carstensen, L. L., Isaacowitz, D. M., & Charles, S. T. (1999). Taking time seriously: A theory of socioemotional selectivity. *American Psychologist, 54,* 165–181.

Casper, L. M., & Bryson, K. R. (1998). *Co-resident grandparents and their grandchildren: Grandparent maintained families* (Population Division Working Paper No. 26). Washington, DC: U.S. Census Bureau.

Cherlin, A. J., & Furstenberg, F. F. (1986). *The new American grandparent: A place in the family, a life apart.* New York: Basic Books.

Crowther, M., & Rodriguez, R. (2003). A stress and coping model of custodial grandparenting among African Americans. In B. Hayslip & J. H. Patrick (Eds.), *Working with custodial grandparents* (pp. 145–162). New York: Springer Publishing Company.

Diener, E., Suh, E., Lucas, R. E., & Smith, H. L. (1999). Subjective well-being: Three decades of progress. *Psychological Bulletin, 125,* 276–302.

Emick, M., & Hayslip, B. (1996). Custodial grandparenting: New roles for middle aged and older adults. *International Journal of Aging and Human Development, 43,* 135–154.

Fields, J., & Casper, L. M. (2001). *America's families and living arrangements: 2000 Current Population Reports* (P20-537). Washington, DC: U.S. Census Bureau. Retrieved March 24, 2005, from http://www.census.gov/prod/2001pubs/p20-537.pdf

Fuller-Thomson, E., & Minkler, M. (2000). The mental and physical health of grandmothers who are raising their grandchildren. *Journal of Mental Health and Aging, 6,* 311–323.

Generations United. (2000). *Grandparents and other relatives raising children: Challenges of caring for the second family: Generations United Fact Sheet.* Retrieved October 3, 2001, from http://www.gu.org/Files/gpgeneral.pdf

Goldberg-Glen, R., & Sands, R. (2000). Primary and secondary caregiving grandparents: How different are they? In B. Hayslip & R. S. Goldberg-Glen (Eds.), *Grandparents raising grandchildren: Theoretical, empirical, and clinical perspectives* (pp. 161–180). New York: Springer Publishing Company.

Goodman, C. C. (2006). Grandmothers raising grandchildren: The vulnerability of advancing age. In B. Hayslip & J. Patrick (Eds.), *Custodial grandparenting: Individual, cultural, and ethnic diversity* (pp. 133–150). New York: Springer Publishing Company.

Hayslip, B. (2003). The impact of a psychosocial intervention on parental efficacy, grandchild relationship quality, and well-being among grandparents raising grandchildren. In B. Hayslip & J. Patrick (Eds.), *Working with custodial grandparents* (pp. 163–178). New York: Springer Publishing Company.

Hayslip, B., Baird, A., Toledo, R., Toledo, C., & Emick, M. (2006). Cross-cultural differences in traditional and custodial grandparenting: A qualitative approach. In B. Hayslip & J. Patrick (Eds.), *Custodial grandparenting: Individual, cultural, and ethnic diversity* (pp. 169–182). New York: Springer Publishing Company.

Hayslip, B., Kaminski, P. L., & Earnheart, K. L. (2006). Gender differences among custodial grandparents. In B. Hayslip & J. H. Patrick (Eds.), *Custodial grandparenting: Individual, cultural, and ethnic diversity* (pp. 151–166). New York: Springer Publishing Company.

Hayslip, B., & Patrick, J. H. (2003). Custodial grandparenting viewed from within a lifespan perspective. In B. Hayslip & J. H. Patrick (Eds.), *Working with custodial grandparents* (pp. 3–11). New York: Springer Publishing Company.

Hayslip, B., Shore, R. J., & Emick, M. A. (2006). Age, health, and custodial grandparenting. In B. Hayslip & J. H. Patrick (Eds.), *Custodial grandparenting: Individual, cultural, and ethnic diversity* (pp. 75–87). New York: Springer Publishing Company.

Hayslip, B., Shore, R. J., & Lambert, P. (1998). Custodial grandparenting and grandchildren with problems: Their impact on role satisfaction and role meaning. *Journal of Gerontology: Social Sciences, 53B,* S164–S174.

Hayslip, B., Temple, J. R., Shore, R. J., & Henderson, C. E. (2006). Determinants of role satisfaction among traditional and custodial grandparents. In B. Hayslip & J. H. Patrick (Eds.), *Custodial grandparenting: Individual, cultural, and ethnic diversity* (pp. 21–36). New York: Springer Publishing Company.

Joslin, D., & Brouard, A. (1995). The prevalence of grandmothers as primary caregivers in a poor pediatric population. *Journal of Community Health, 20,* 383–401

Karp, N. (1996). Legal problems of grandparents and other kinship caregivers. *Generations, 20,* 57–60.

Kern, C. W. (2003). Grandparents who are parenting again: Building parenting skills. In B. Hayslip & J. H. Patrick (Eds.), *Working with custodial grandparents* (pp. 179–193). New York: Springer Publishing Company.

Kinney, J. M., McGrew, K. B., & Nelson, I. M. (2003). Grandparent caregivers to children with developmental disabilities: Added challenges. In B. Hayslip & J. H. Patrick (Eds.), *Working with custodial grandparents* (pp. 93–109). New York: Springer Publishing Company.

Kohn, S. J., & Smith, G. C. (2006). Social support among custodial grandparents within a diversity of contexts. In B. Hayslip & J. H. Patrick (Eds.), *Custodial grandparenting: Individual, cultural, and ethnic diversity* (pp. 199–223). New York: Springer Publishing Company.

Kolomer, S. R. (2000). Kinship foster care and its impact on grandmother caregivers. *Journal of Gerontological Social Work, 33,* 85–102.

Lazarus, R. S., & Folkman, S. (1984). *Stress, appraisals, and coping.* New York: Springer Publishing Company.

Lee, R. D., Ensminger, M. E., & LaVeist, T. A. (2006). African-American grandmothers: The responsibility continuum. In B. Hayslip & J. H. Patrick (Eds.), *Custodial grandparenting: Individual, cultural, and ethnic diversity* (pp. 119–132). New York: Springer Publishing Company.

Lee, S., Colditz, G., Berkman, L., & Kawachi, I. (2003). Caregiving to children and grandchildren and risk of coronary heart disease in women. *American Journal of Public Health, 93,* 1939–1944.

Lerner, R. (1996). *Concepts and theories of human development.* New York: Random House.

Mackintosh, V. H., Myers, B. J., & Kennon, S. S. (2006). Children of incarcerated mothers and their caregivers: Factors affecting the quality of their relationship. *Journal of Child and Family Studies, 15,* 581–596.

McCallion, P., & Kolomer, S. R. (2006). Depression and caregiver mastery in grandfathers caring for their grandchildren. In B. Hayslip & J. H. Patrick (Eds.), *Custodial grandparenting: Individual, cultural, and ethnic diversity* (pp. 105–118). New York: Springer Publishing Company.

McGowen, M. R., Ladd, L., & Strom, R. D. (2006). On-line assessment of grandmother experience in raising grandchildren. *Educational Gerontology, 32,* 669–684.

Minkler, M., Fuller-Thomson, E., Miller, D., & Driver, D. (1997). Depression in grandparents raising grandchildren: Results of a national longitudinal study. *Archives of Family Medicine, 6,* 445–452.

Minkler, M., & Roe, K. M. (1993). *Grandmothers as caregivers: Raising children of the crack cocaine epidemic.* Newbury Park, CA: Sage.

Musil, C. M. (1998). Health, stress, coping, and social support in grandmother caregivers. *Health Care for Women International, 19,* 441–455.

Neugarten, B. L., & Weinstein, K. K. (1964). The changing American grandparent. *Journal of Marriage and the Family, 26,* 199–204.

Patrick, J. H., & Hayden, J. M. (1999). Neuroticism, coping strategies, and negative well-being among caregivers. *Psychology and Aging, 14,* 273–283.

Patrick, J. H., Hayslip, B., & Tomczewski, D. K. (2008). *Emerging adults' attitudes toward custodial grandparents.* Unpublished manuscript, West Virginia University, Morgantown.

Patrick, J. H., & Pickard, J. (2003). Grandmother–grandchild interactions. In B. Hayslip & J. H. Patrick (Eds.), *Working with custodial grandparents* (pp. 229–242). New York: Springer Publishing Company.

4

Patrick, J. H., & Tomczewski, D. K. (2007). Custodial grandfathers. *Journal of Intergenerational Relations, 5*(4), 113–116.

Pruchno, R. (1999). Raising grandchildren: The experiences of Black and White grandmothers. *The Gerontologist, 39,* 209–221.

Pruchno, R., & McKenney, D. (2006). Grandmothers raising grandchildren: The effects of work disruptions on current work. In B. Hayslip & J. Patrick (Eds.), *Custodial grandparenting: Individual, cultural, and ethnic diversity* (pp. 3–20). New York: Springer Publishing Company.

Riegel, K. (1976). The dialectics of human development. *American Psychologist, 31,* 689–700.

Robbins, M. S., Briones, E., Schwartz, S. J., Dillon, F. R., & Mitrani, V. B. (2006). Differences in family functioning in grandparent and parent-headed households in a clinical sample of drug-using African American adolescents. *Cultural Diversity & Ethnic Minority Psychology, 12,* 84–100.

Roberto, K., & Qualls, S. (2003). Intervention strategies for grandparents raising grandchildren: Lessons learned from the late life caregiving literature. In B. Hayslip & J. H. Patrick (Eds.), *Working with custodial grandparents* (pp. 13–26). New York: Springer Publishing Company.

Silverstein, M. (2007). Benefits of grandparents raising grandchildren. *Journal of Intergenerational Relationships, 5,* 131–134.

Simmons, T., & Dye, J. L. (2003). *Grandparents living with grandchildren: 2000.* Retrieved October 14, 2007, from http://www.census.gov/prod/2003pubs/c2kbr-31.pdf

Smith, G. C. (2003). How caregiving grandparents view support groups: An exploratory study. In B. Hayslip & J. H. Patrick (Eds.), *Working with custodial grandparents* (pp. 69–91). New York: Springer Publishing Company.

Solomon, J. C., & Marx, J. (1998). The grandparent–grandchild caregiving gradient: Hours of caring for grandchildren and its relationship to grandparent health. *Southwest Journal of Aging, 14,* 31–39.

Strawbridge, W. J., Wallhagen, M. I., Shema, S. J., & Kaplan, G. A. (1997). New burdens or more of the same? Comparing grandparent, spouse, and adult-child caregivers. *The Gerontologist, 37,* 505–510.

Strom, R. D., & Strom, S. K. (2000). Meeting the challenge of raising grandchildren. *International Journal of Aging and Human Development, 51,* 183–198.

Strough, J., Patrick, J. H., & Swenson, L. (2003). Strategies for solving everyday problems faced by grandparents: The role of experience. In B. Hayslip & J. H. Patrick (Eds.), *Working with custodial grandparents* (pp. 257–275). New York: Springer Publishing Company.

Szinovacz, M. E. (1998). Grandparents today: A demographic profile. *The Gerontologist, 38,* 37–52.

Szinovacz, M. E., & Davey, A. (2006). Effects of retirement and grandchild care on depressive symptoms. *International Journal of Aging and Human Development, 62,* 1–20.

Thomas, J. L. (1989). Gender and perceptions of grandparenthood. *International Journal of Aging and Human Development, 29,* 269–282.

Troll, L. E. (1985). The contingencies of grandparenting. In V. L. Bengtson & J. F. Roberts (Eds.), *Grandparenthood* (pp. 135–149). Beverly Hills, CA: Sage.

U.S. Census Bureau. (2005). *American Community Survey.* Retrieved December 1, 2007, from http://www.census.gov/acs/www/index.html

Wang, Y., & Marcotte, D. E. (2007, February). *Golden years? The labor market effects of caring for grandchildren.* (Institute for the Study of Labor Discussion Paper No. 2629). Bonn, Germany: Institute for the Study of Labor.

Winokur, M., Rozen, D., Thompson, S., Green, S., & Valentine, D. (2005). *Kinship care in the United States: A systematic review of evidence-based research: Final Report.* Fort Collins: Colorado State University.

Young, M. H., & Dawson, T. J. (2003). Perception of child difficulty and levels of depression in caregiving grandmothers. *Journal of Mental Health & Aging, 9,* 111–122.

Afterword

Kim Shifren

This volume has covered the theoretical and empirical research on caregiving throughout the life span, from caregivers in childhood through grandparent caregivers. Each contributor has described caregiving by using the life span development framework, which involves the ideas that development is (a) lifelong, (b) dependent on history and context, (c) multidimensional and multidirectional, and (d) pliable (Baltes, Lindenberger, & Staudinger, 1998). Developmental tasks that are part of normal development have been discussed, and whenever data were available, comparisons between caregiving and noncaregiving samples on these tasks were provided.

The gains and losses that occur as a result of caregiving experiences across developmental periods have been discussed. *Gains*, or positive effects of caregiving, have been demonstrated for each developmental period assessed. In chapter 1, Bauman and colleagues found that caregivers in middle childhood and adolescence who provided emotional support to parents did not have higher depression than those who did not provide this support. Those who took on caregiver roles tended to have higher scores on parent–child relationship scales than those who did not. In chapter 3, Dellmann-Jenkins and Blankemeyer found that compared with the noncaregiving sample, emerging or young adult caregivers have close relations with care recipients, better self-respect, and autonomy. In chapter 5, Stephens and colleagues found that juggling the parent-care and work roles is complex, as would be expected from the life span approach, and that well-being can be maintained when positive experiences from one role buffer against negative effects of the other role. In chapter 6, Patrick and Goedereis found that older grandmothers suffered less distress from providing care to grandchildren than younger grandmothers.

Losses also have been documented for each developmental period. For example, in chapter 1, Bauman and colleagues found that middle childhood and adolescent caregivers who provided regular amounts of personal care had more behavior problems. In chapter 2, Siskowski found that almost half of adolescent caregivers in the What Works Survey reported that caregiving hindered learning, and this was more likely to be true for boys than girls and for older rather than younger adolescents. From a life span perspective, the complex changes taking place during adolescence may interact with the caregiving experience, leading to more challenges for the adolescent caregiver than are present for the caregiver in middle childhood. In chapter 6, Patrick and Goedereis found that grandparent caregivers have reported more depressive symptoms and more stress if they provide full-time rather than part-time care for grandchildren and that grandmother caregivers have worse physical health than noncaregiver samples. Much like the results in chapter 1 on the youngest caregivers, the oldest caregivers show gender differences. Grandfathers tend to have more depressive symptoms and more disruptions because of providing child care than grandmothers. These gender differences might be explained by different socialization practices in our society; throughout history, different behaviors and jobs for males and females have been shaped and modeled (Shifren, Furnham, & Bauserman, 1998).

Whether the overall balance in the effects of caregiving is negative or positive depends on the context in which caregivers live. Those who view caregiving as nonnormative tend to experience more losses or negative effects of caregiving over time than those who view caregiving as a normal part of life. As I discussed in the introduction to this volume, chapters 1 and 6 show that race can play an important role in caregiver experiences. African American caregivers provide more care than Caucasian caregivers but find the experience less stressful and disruptive.

Regardless of the developmental period of the caregiver discussed, the overall evidence presented throughout this book shows that mental health problems are not inevitable. Even caregivers in childhood who provide care to their parents show evidence of positive effects from their caregiving experiences (see chap. 1).

As we have seen, caregiving can begin and end at any time in the life span and is characterized by an ongoing interaction between the caregiving role and development. This supports the idea of lifelong development as an ongoing dynamic (Baltes et al., 1998). Recent history is notable for the advancements that have led to increased life spans and changes in family composition. Caregivers can be very young and very old, and they take on roles that were not required of earlier generations. Historical context thus plays a role in developmental processes.

Research summarized in this book includes sample participants from unique contexts and demonstrates how context affects development. For example, a study comparing inner city mothers with HIV/AIDS and their children with a noncaregiving group was summarized in chapter 1; a survey of adolescents from Palm Beach County, Florida, that included a large proportion of Hispanic respondents was described in chapter 2; and research involving samples more representative of middle-class Americans was discussed in chapters 3 and 4.

Multiple dimensions are involved in human development. Both caregivers' and noncaregivers' development involves physical, cognitive, and psychosocial changes throughout the life span. This book has touched on some of the physical changes that occur in adolescence (chap. 2) and in middle-aged and older adults (chaps. 5 and 6). The majority of research described in the book focused on psychosocial changes in the development of caregivers, including parentification, filial responsibility, and felt obligation. In addition, the effects of juggling caregiving and work roles as well as dealing with work and retirement issues along with grandparent caregiving roles were examined.

It should be clear from this book that the caregiving experience is complex. Although it may be impossible to capture a body of research as large as caregiving under one theoretical model, the life span development framework can be used as a consistent theoretical view across different periods of development.

DIRECTIONS FOR FUTURE RESEARCH

The use of the life span development theoretical framework can help researchers formulate future studies encompassing all of the caregiving age groups across the life span. Here, I touch on a number of issues that could be addressed in such research.

Questions of Interest

Child and Adolescent Caregivers

Much additional investigation is needed of the very youngest caregivers in the United States. Many questions are of interest, but only a few are provided here to exemplify the work that needs to be done:

1. For whom do young caregivers provide care (e.g., mothers, fathers, sisters, brothers, aunts, uncles, grandparents)?
2. How does providing help for siblings, parents, and others in activities of daily living affect children's mental and physical health currently and over the life span?
3. Can theoretical models of adult coping and stress be applied to child and adolescent caregivers?
4. In terms of research on filial responsibility and felt obligation, will the youngest caregivers have the most filial responsibility or felt obligation compared with other groups? Why or why not?
5. How does the role of personality affect caregivers' perceptions and decisions regarding the caregiving situation as well as friendship networks and school attendance and performance?
6. How might the reduced time for building social relationships in childhood and adolescence that is a result of taking on the caregiving role influence child and adolescent caregivers' well-being in adulthood? Are they at a disadvantage for building their social networks into adulthood?

Emerging and Young Adult Caregivers

More research is also needed on emerging and young adult caregivers. The following are among the questions to pursue for this age range:

1. How does caregiving in emerging and young adulthood affect the individuals' current and future mental and physical health?
2. Can the coping and stress models from the older adult caregiving literature be useful for studying and explaining behavior in this age group?
3. How do limited social activities and time in this age group relate to future well-being?

Middle Adult Caregivers

Women and men are marrying and having babies at later ages. This poses new questions for middle adult caregivers:

1. Is simultaneous caregiving for very young children and one's parents significantly different from caregiving for older children and one's parents? Why or why not?
2. What are the obstacles that women and men in middle adulthood face when providing care for others? How do these compare with obstacles faced by previous generations?
3. How might the trend toward having babies later in life affect one's ability to work, both inside and outside of the home, while performing caregiving tasks?

Older Caregivers

Although research on grandparent caregivers in the middle and older adult developmental periods has increased, many questions remain to be answered·

1. What is it like for a great-grandparent to provide care to babies and small children?

2. How might living in or near multigeneration families (great-grandchildren and great-grandparents) affect the dynamics of the caregiving role?

3. Will grandchildren and great-grandchildren provide care for their grandparents and great-grandparents at an increased rate over time?

4. Will the older adult caregiver provide care for relatives who can live longer and longer with chronic health problems over increasing periods of time?

Study Design Issues

Diversity

One consistent theme that emerges across the chapters in this book is the need for larger and more diverse sampling of socioeconomic status, employment types, geographic location, family structure, and culture and ethnicity. Sampling a wider socioeconomic status range is important because of the effects this variable has on education, health care access, support availability, nutrition, and overall quality of life. Caregiving in the context of poverty is much different from caregiving in a middle-class context, and middle-class families have experiences that may not reflect the experiences of the elite of our society. What kinds of caregiving issues face the very wealthy in the United States? Are the issues faced by the very wealthy similar to or different from those faced by the rest of society?

Types of employment are also important in research about caregiving. Some jobs provide flexible days and work hours, which enable caregivers to juggle caregiving and employment responsibilities, whereas other jobs do not. Obviously, a society in which individuals increasingly assume caregiving responsibilities for older family members and sick younger members requires a workforce that reflects the need to fulfill these roles. Will there be significant changes in the type of leave available at work and flexibility in scheduling time? How will changes or the lack of them affect caregiving experiences?

Geographic location is not often a focus of caregiving research, but different geographic locations may affect the caregiving experience. Individuals in warmer climates may find it easier to do the errands necessary to maintain a household with a care recipient. Individuals in colder climates may have limited access to pharmacies, grocery stores, and hospitals during severe weather conditions. Even everyday experiences such as going for walks with the care recipient or by oneself, which may be taken for granted in warmer climates, are sometimes not available in colder climates. Individuals who live in rural regions tend to be more isolated and farther from medical resources than those in suburban or urban areas.

Family structure appears to play an important role in the perceptions and decisions of young people to become caregivers for family members or friends (Dellmann-Jenkins, Blankemeyer, & Pinkard, 2001; Shifren, 2008; Stein et al., 1998). Future studies should provide comparisons between caregiving by single-parent and intact (i.e., in which parents are married and living together) families and noncaregiving groups and between sole- and joint-custody (legal and physical custody) arrangements. The presence of one versus two parents in the household is an important issue not only for child caregivers but for caregivers in other age groups as well. How do single-parent families compare with intact families over the life span in terms of caregiving experiences? Are experiences significantly different between each age group or do differences disappear as people get older? Are there significant differences in the caregiving experiences of individuals from sole- versus joint-custody families, and do the differences remain over time? Do multigenerational families live together or near each other now that people are living longer? How might the presence of very young and very old individuals in the same household affect the caregiving experiences of child, adolescent, emerging adult, and young adult caregivers compared with middle and older adult caregivers? Are the caregiving experiences of same-sex versus heterosexual couples the same or different?

It is also important to address cultural and ethnic similarities and differences in caregiving research, and there is clearly a need for further examination of these variables in future studies. The role of culture and ethnicity in caregiving from a life span perspective is important because the timing of developmental tasks appears to differ by ethnicity (U.S. Census Bureau, 2003). Although some research has been conducted to assess ethnic and cultural differences in middle and older adult caregivers (Lum, 2005), little work has been done in this area for the emerging and young adult caregiver groups (for an exception, see Freeberg & Stein, 1996). The child and adolescent caregiver groups presented in this book provide both ethnically and culturally diverse samples. However, these studies are the first of their kind, and additional studies are certainly warranted for replication purposes. All developmental periods would benefit from the inclusion of more diverse samples of caregivers.

Ethical Issues

Researchers cannot ethically conduct a scientific study on child and adolescent caregivers and simply walk away. We must prepare our studies in a way that enables young caregivers to find help by directing participants to available resources such as support groups and health services. Even studies focused on basic research questions need to provide direction in locating resources to help young caregivers when participants have completed the study. Providing assistance can be something as simple as distributing a list of local resources with contact information for support groups, health care services, financial assistance information, and school tutors. Adults who receive care from children may also find themselves in difficult situations; researchers who come across such situations have an ethical obligation to suggest ways to provide support, if possible.

Longitudinal Studies

Authors in this volume have discussed the need to conduct longitudinal studies. Caregiving research from the life span perspective necessarily involves performing longitudinal studies, beginning in childhood and continuing through older adulthood, to determine the effects of caregiving on multiple aspects of development within caregivers as they age. It is important to understand both short- and long-term effects of caregiving on the caregiver, and cross-sectional research cannot address this issue. Cross-sectional studies may involve cohort effects that cannot be easily separated from age differences found in samples of caregivers

(Papalia, Olds, & Feldman, 2007). Ideally, nationwide studies could be conducted on random samples of households with assessments every 3 to 5 years throughout the life span. This would help determine who becomes a caregiver and how early the caregiving role really starts. It would also provide better understanding of the effects of caregiving over the life span.

CONCLUSION

I have raised here just some of the possible questions of interest for future research on caregiving using a life span framework. I hope that they will also stimulate thinking about additional questions as well as planning for more ambitious future research. Multiple longitudinal studies that address any and all of the above questions about caregiving over the life span, incorporating the role of history and context and the multidimensional aspects of individuals when discussing gains and losses in caregiver development, would be of great value to the caregiving literature.

REFERENCES

Baltes, P. B., Lindenberger, U., & Staudinger, U. M. (1998). Life-span theory in developmental psychology. In R. M. Lerner (Ed.), *Handbook of child psychology: Vol. 1. Theoretical models of human development* (pp. 1029–1143). New York: Wiley.

Dellmann-Jenkins, M., Blankemeyer, M., & Pinkard, O. (2001). Incorporating the elder caregiving role into the developmental tasks of young adulthood. *Journal of Aging and Human Development, 52,* 1–18.

Freeberg, A. L., & Stein, C. H. (1996). Felt obligations towards parents in Mexican-American and Anglo-American young adults. *Journal of Social and Personal Relationships, 13,* 457–471.

Lum, T. Y. (2005). Understanding the racial and ethnic differences in caregiving arrangements. *Journal of Gerontological Social Work, 45,* 3–21.

Papalia, D. E., Olds, S. W., & Feldman, R. D. (2007). *Human development* (10th ed.). New York: McGraw-Hill.

Shifren, K. (2008). *Early caregiving: Perceived parental relations and current social support.* Manuscript under review.

Shifren, K., Furnham, A., & Bauserman, R. L. (1998). Instrumental and expressive traits and eating attitudes: A replication across American and British students. *Personality and Individual Differences, 25,* 1–17.

Stein, C. H., Wemmerus, V.A., Ward, M., Gaines, M. E., Freeberg, A. L., & Jewell, T. C. (1998). "Because they're my parents": An intergenerational study of felt obligation and parental care giving. *Journal of Marriage and Family, 60,* 611–622.

U.S. Census Bureau. (2003, October). *Grandparents living with grandchildren: 2000. Census 2000 brief.* Retrieved April 14, 2008, from http://www.census. gov/prod/2003pubs/c2kbr-31.pdf

Author Index

Page numbers in italics refer to listings in the references.

Wang, R. F., 112, *115*
Wang, Y., 176, 179, 180, *190*
Ward, M., *34, 117,* 128, *145, 200*
Ward, R., 97, *117*
Warner, L., 77, *88*
Watkins, S. C., 119, 132, *145*
Webb, A., *63, 90*
Weinstein, K. K., 169, *188*
Weiss, C. O., 26, *35*
Welsh, R. C., *33*
Wemmerus, V. A., *34, 117,* 122, *145, 200*
Wethington, E., 159, *167*
Wheatley, S. M., 17, *30*
White, L., 97, *117*
White-Means, S. J., 23, *35*
Whitlatch, C. J., 156, *164*
Williams, D., 7, 27, *30*

Williams, S. W., 67, *88, 91*
Williamson, J., 60, *62*
Willis, S. L., 22, *35,* 94, *116*
Winokur, M., 182, *190*
Wojno, W. C., 26, *33*
Wolff, J. L., 93, 104, *117,* 149, 150, 156, 157, *167*
Wolfsen, C., 103, *117*
Woodbury, S., 156, *166*
Worsham, N. L., 69, 86, *91*

Yee, J. L., 11, *35,* 84, *91*
Yoder, A. E., 18, *35*
Young, M. H., 175, 177, *190*

Zacks, R. T., 25, *35*
Zarit, S. H., 3, *33,* 156, *164*
Zhang, J., 3, *35*

Subject Index

About the Editor

Kim Shifren, PhD, earned her bachelor's degree from the University of Maryland, Baltimore County, Catonsville, in 1988, where she majored in psychology with a concentration in biopsychology and minored in sociology. She then went on to receive her master of arts and PhD in life span developmental psychology from Syracuse University, Syracuse, New York, in 1991 and 1993, respectively, under the mentorship of Karen Hooker. Before defending her dissertation, Dr. Shifren became a visiting assistant professor of psychology at the University of Florida, Gainesville. She held this position from 1993 through 1996, and then she began a postdoctoral fellowship at the Institute of Gerontology at the University of Michigan, Ann Arbor, in 1996, with her postdoctoral mentor, Denise Park. Dr. Shifren moved from the Institute of Gerontology to the Institute of Social Research with Park's research group and remained there until the end of her postdoctoral fellowship in 1998. She began a tenure-track position in the Department of Psychology at Towson University, Towson, Maryland, in 1998, and she received tenure and promotion to associate professor in 2003.